Family Values and Social Justice

In making the argument for the remedy of inequality, contemporary political philosophers often emphasize the arbitrariness of disadvantage, stressing how one's lot in life is to a significant extent determined by the circumstances of one's birth, that is, in which family, and in what part of the world. In the latter instance, people differ in how well they live in a large part because of their context in the global order. But equally important for a person's chances in life is the family that raises her (if the person is lucky enough to have a family in the first place). In *Family Values: The Ethics of Parent-Child Relationships,* Harry Brighouse and Adam Swift provide a systematic analysis of the morality and politics of the family, exploring why families are valuable, whether people have a right to parent, what rights and duties parents have, and, in particular, what rights children have that may constrain the rights of their parents. The essays in this volume assess Brighouse and Swift's contribution, taking up a number of controversial issues about autonomy, human flourishing, parental rights, and indeed the nature of childhood itself. Contributors offer a range of arguments, some challenging, others complementing, of Brighouse and Swift's account of the ethics of parent-child relationships.

The chapters in this book were originally published in a special issue of the *Critical Review of International Social and Political Philosophy.*

Andrée-Anne Cormier is an Assistant Professor of Philosophy at York University, Glendon College, Toronto, Canada. She was previously a postdoctoral fellow in the Law Department at the Universitat Pompeu Fabra, Barcelona, Spain, where she worked as a member of the Family Justice research project, funded by the European Research Council. Her current research focuses primarily on issues of legitimacy in upbringing, childhood, and gender justice. She also has published articles in philosophy of education and animal ethics.

Christine Sypnowich is a Professor, a Queen's National Scholar, and the Head of Philosophy at Queen's University, Kingston, Canada. She is the author of *Equality Renewed: Justice, Flourishing and the Egalitarian Ideal* (Routledge, 2016) and *The Concept of Socialist Law* (1990), editor of *The Egalitarian Conscience: Essays in Honour of G.A. Cohen* (2006), and co-editor (with David Bakhurst) of *The Social Self* (1995). She is currently working on a book on G.A. Cohen, as well as starting a new project on heritage and political philosophy. Her work has appeared in such journals as *Political Theory, Oxford Journal of Legal Studies, New Left Review,* and *Politics and Society.*

Family Values and Social Justice

Reflections on *Family Values: the Ethics of Parent-Child Relationships* by H. Brighouse and A. Swift

Edited by
Andrée-Anne Cormier and Christine Sypnowich

Routledge
Taylor & Francis Group
LONDON AND NEW YORK

First published 2019
by Routledge
2 Park Square, Milton Park, Abingdon, Oxon, OX14 4RN, UK

and by Routledge
52 Vanderbilt Avenue, New York, NY 10017, USA

First issued in paperback 2020

Routledge is an imprint of the Taylor & Francis Group, an informa business

British Library Cataloguing-in-Publication Data
A catalogue record for this book is available from the British Library

ISBN 13: 978-0-367-58615-7 (pbk)
ISBN 13: 978-1-138-33072-6 (hbk)

Typeset in Myriad Pro
by codeMantra

Publisher's Note
The publisher accepts responsibility for any inconsistencies that may have arisen during the conversion of this book from journal articles to book chapters, namely the possible inclusion of journal terminology.

Contents

Citation Information

The chapters in this book were originally published in the journal *Critical Review of International Social and Political Philosophy*, volume 21, issue 3 (June 2018). When citing this material, please use the original page numbering for each article, as follows:

Introduction
Andrée-Anne Cormier and Christine Sypnowich
Critical Review of International Social and Political Philosophy, volume 21, issue 3 (June 2018) pp. 279–283

Chapter 1
What abolishing the family would not do
Anca Gheaus
Critical Review of International Social and Political Philosophy, volume 21, issue 3 (June 2018) pp. 284–300

Chapter 2
Equality and family values: conflict or harmony?
Colin M. Macleod
Critical Review of International Social and Political Philosophy, volume 21, issue 3 (June 2018) pp. 301–313

Chapter 3
Flourishing children, flourishing adults: families, equality and the neutralism-perfectionism debate
Christine Sypnowich
Critical Review of International Social and Political Philosophy, volume 21, issue 3 (June 2018) pp. 314–332

Chapter 4

On the permissibility of shaping children's values
Andrée-Anne Cormier
Critical Review of International Social and Political Philosophy, volume 21, issue 3 (June 2018) pp. 333–350

Chapter 5

For a political philosophy of parent–child relationships
Daniel Weinstock
Critical Review of International Social and Political Philosophy, volume 21, issue 3 (June 2018) pp. 351–365

Chapter 6

Childhood bads, parenting goods, and the right to procreate
Sarah Hannan and R. J. Leland
Critical Review of International Social and Political Philosophy, volume 21, issue 3 (June 2018) pp. 366–384

Chapter 7

Family values reconsidered: a response
Harry Brighouse and Adam Swift
Critical Review of International Social and Political Philosophy, volume 21, issue 3 (June 2018) pp. 385–405

Notes on Contributors

Harry Brighouse is a Professor of Philosophy, Carol Dickson-Bascom Professor of the Humanities, an Affiliate Professor of Educational Policy Studies, and Director of the Center for Ethics and Education at the University of Wisconsin-Madison, USA. His interests include political philosophy, philosophy of education, and education policy.

Andrée-Anne Cormier is an Assistant Professor of Philosophy at York University, Glendon College, Toronto, Canada. Her current research focuses primarily on issues of legitimacy in upbringing, childhood, and gender justice. She also has published articles in philosophy of education and animal ethics.

Anca Gheaus is a Ramon y Cajal Researcher at the Pompeu Fabra University, Barcelona, Spain. She has published numerous articles on family ethics and various aspects of distributive justice in publications such as the *Journal of Political Philosophy*, the *Philosophical Quarterly*, the *Journal of Applied Philosophy*, and the *Journal of Medical Ethics*.

Sarah Hannan is an Assistant Professor of Political Studies at the University of Manitoba, Winnipeg, Canada. Her research is in moral and political philosophy. She has published articles in *Theory and Research in Education* (2008) and the *Journal of Applied Philosophy* (2017). She is the co-editor of *Permissible Progeny?: The Morality of Procreation and Parenting* (with Samantha Brennan and Richard Vernon, 2015).

R. J. Leland is an Assistant Professor of Philosophy at the University of Manitoba, Winnipeg, Canada. His research is in moral and political philosophy. His work has appeared in *Ethics* (2012), *The Journal of Moral Philosophy* (2017), and *Philosophy and Phenomenological Research* (2017).

Colin M. Macleod is a Professor of Philosophy and Law at the University of Victoria, Canada. His research focuses on issues in contemporary moral, political, and legal theory with a special focus on distributive justice and equality; children, families, and justice; and democratic ethics. His work includes *Liberalism, Justice, and Markets* (1998) and *The Moral and Political Status of Children* (co-edited with David Archard, 2002).

Adam Swift is a Professor in the Department of Political Science at University College, London, UK. At the time of writing, his most recent book (with Harry Brighouse, Helen F. Ladd, and Susanna Loeb) is *Educational Goods: Values, Evidence and Decision Making* (2018).

Christine Sypnowich is a Professor, a Queen's National Scholar, and the Head of Philosophy at Queen's University, Kingston, Canada. She is the author of *Equality Renewed: Justice, Flourishing and the Egalitarian Ideal* (Routledge, 2016) and *The Concept of Socialist Law* (1990), editor of *The Egalitarian Conscience: Essays in Honour of G.A. Cohen* (2006), and co-editor (with David Bakhurst) of *The Social Self* (1995).

Daniel Weinstock is a Professor in the Faculty of Law at McGill University, Montreal, Canada, where he also directs the Institute for Health and Social Policy. He has written extensively on the ethics and politics of childhood and the family.

Introduction

Andrée-Anne Cormier and Christine Sypnowich

In making the argument for the remedy of inequality, contemporary political philosophers often emphasize the arbitrariness of disadvantage. There are many ways in which inequality results from factors beyond people's control. To take two striking examples, one's lot in life is to a significant extent determined by where one is born, that is, in which family, and in what part of the world. In the latter instance, people differ in how well they live in large part because of their context in the global order, that is, if they live in a well off or impoverished part of the world, if there are just or unjust institutions, a tolerant or repressive culture. But equally important for a person's chances in life is the family that raises her (if the person is lucky enough to have a family in the first place). It matters whether the family has material resources and how much, whether parents have good or bad parenting skills, are supportive or neglectful, or have sufficient opportunities to care for their children. And just as one cannot choose what part of the world to be born in, one cannot choose which family to raise one to adulthood. Moreover, these two sources of arbitrary advantage and disadvantage intersect, since some countries in the world have well-developed social welfare institutions to support families and the raising of children, and thereby mitigate the contingencies of family circumstances, while elsewhere these contingencies are untouched or worsened by a society's practices. It is thus appropriate that political philosophy, for so long focused on the policies of (largely Western) nations, has recently extended its scope in order to tackle the macro issues of global justice, and the micro issues of familial justice.

Harry Brighouse and Adam Swift have contributed an important work of scholarship on the latter question. *Family Values: the Ethics of Parent-Child Relationships* provides a systematic analysis of the morality and politics of the family, exploring why families are valuable, whether people have a right to parent, what rights and duties parents have, and in particular what rights children have that may constrain the rights of their parents. The book focuses on a number of conflicting moral imperatives. At the heart of the book is the idea that parent–child relationships produce the familial relationship goods that enable children, and also parents, to flourish. Children's healthy development depends on intimate relationships with authoritative adults, while the distinctive joys and challenges of parenting are part of a fulfilling life for many adults. Brighouse and Swift explore why a child's interest in autonomy significantly limits parents' right to deliberately try to shape their children's values, and why parents have no fundamental right to confer wealth or advantage on their children. The book reaffirms the vital importance of the family as a social institution while challenging its role in the reproduction of social inequality, and making the case for carefully balancing the interests of parents and children. The book's complex argument raises a number of controversial issues about autonomy, human flourishing, parental rights, and indeed the nature of childhood itself. The essays of this volume consider these issues and offer a range of arguments and considerations, some challenging and others complementing Brighouse and Swift's account of the ethics of parent-child relationships.

Anca Gheaus's paper challenges one key assumption endorsed by most family justice theorists in the liberal egalitarian tradition, namely, that the family undermines equality of opportunity and other fair patterns of distribution in some special sort of way, as John Rawls famously commented. According to Gheaus, Brighouse and Swift take for granted this basic claim about the special tension between equality of opportunity and the family. In her view, however, there is reason to resist such a claim. Gheaus's central idea is that although the family does indeed disrupt fair patterns of distribution, and equality of opportunity in particular, alternative childrearing arrangements would also be disruptive in similar ways, and for similar reasons. This is so because the key elements that undermine equality of opportunity – caregivers' partiality toward specific children and their unequal ability to provide good care – 'go deeper' than the family itself. They would be present in any other decent childrearing institution. Furthermore, Gheaus suggests, the institution of the family is not the only social mechanism that allows for the accumulation of economic inequalities. She concludes that family justice theorists should simply abandon the project of addressing Rawls's famous (perhaps rhetorical?) question as to why the family should not be abolished in the name of equality. Since any acceptable alternative to the family would similarly disrupt equality of opportunity, liberal egalitarians should not devote much intellectual energy to justifying the family against possible (unattainable and all-things-considered less desirable) alternatives.

Like Gheaus, Colin M. Macleod focuses primarily on the issue of the presumed tension between equality of opportunity and the family. Macleod also denies that abolishing the family would in fact advance equality of opportunity. His paper's main suggestion, however, is not that alternatives to the family would potentially disrupt equality of opportunity in similar ways (although he appears to agree with Gheaus on this point), but rather that there is no inevitable conflict between family values and equality of opportunity – contrary to what he takes Brighouse and Swift to believe. More precisely, in a suitably non-hierarchical (ideal) society, familial relationship goods could be realized at no cost to egalitarian justice. The main argumentative strategy deployed by Macleod consists in challenging key claims which he takes to ground the idea of a principled 'ineliminable tension' between familial relationship goods and equality of opportunity. In particular, Macleod suggests, in an idealized egalitarian political community, differences in terms of parental abilities and the development of valuable skills in children would be rather negligible, both as a result of egalitarian social arrangements and because well-functioning institutions would mitigate the residual differences effectively.

Christine Sypnowich's paper explores another, rather different, set of issues. She takes the authors to task for failing to appreciate fully the perfectionist implications of their position. Political philosophers are divided on the question of whether society should guide individuals to improve their wellbeing. *Family Values,* however, affirms that the flourishing of children requires relationships in which parents also flourish; and that furthermore, parents' flourishing is itself a reason to safeguard the relationship goods of the family. Yet, Sypnowich notes that Brighouse and Swift are concerned that their position be compatible with liberal neutralist accounts wherein the state does not seek to promote valuable ways of living. She contends, however, that once we see the role of the family in enabling the flourishing of children, we cannot avoid a commitment to furthering human flourishing more generally. The argument about the rearing and education of children falls down, Sypnowich argues, unless it presupposes a fact of the matter – however, pluralistic and non-coercive – about living well and the proper role of the state in promoting it. After all, she contends, we need to identify what adult flourishing looks like in order to equip children for it, and we need to provide conditions to ensure that children, upon maturation, will be able to actualize their capacities to live well. Moreover, on her 'egalitarian flourishing' account, a public commitment to providing support so that families may thrive can be seen as an equalizing policy. Sypnowich concludes that Brighouse and Swift's powerful argument for why families are valuable, and the intrinsically valuable relationship goods rightly enjoyed by all their members, makes it clear that political philosophy has been impoverished for its jettisoning of questions of human flourishing. Once we understand the flourishing provided by families, we should be prepared to develop an egalitarian political philosophy that centers on enabling flourishing, more broadly, for all.

Andrée-Anne Cormier's paper examines a related issue concerning liberal neutrality or anti-perfectionism in upbringing, but from a rather different perspective. Her paper addresses the question of whether, and under what conditions, it is permissible for parents deliberately to try to shape their children's particular comprehensive values in light of their own. She offers an extended defense of the view endorsed by Brighouse and Swift that at least some forms of deliberate comprehensive value-shaping are permissible. This is in opposition to Matthew Clayton's challenging account of legitimate childrearing, according to which the deliberate shaping of children's values is impermissible in principle, since it violates a principle of respect for children's independence. Drawing on Brighouse and Swift's account of familial relationship goods, Cormier suggests that seeking to pass on comprehensive values to one's child is in fact compatible with proper respect for the child's independence, as Clayton understands it. This is because at least some limited forms of deliberate parental value-shaping can pass what she takes to be the most plausible test of respect for children's independence, namely, the 'anti-perfectionist test of retrospective consent'.

Daniel Weinstock's essay focuses on 'the juggling act between intimacy and autonomy' that appears to daunt family life. On the one hand, parents and children share valuable relationship goods; on the other hand, those very goods can act to undermine children's ability to choose for themselves how their lives will go. And, though it is easy to pinpoint when it is illegitimate for parents to confer socioeconomic advantages, it is much harder to isolate impermissible forms of value-sharing. This is because, as Weinstock puts it, the difference between permissible and impermissible ways of sharing conceptions of the good with one's children is, on the *Family Values* account, 'adverbial' rather than 'categorical'. In other words, it is the manner in which values are shared, rather than the fact of value sharing itself, which requires monitoring. But value-sharing is so bound up with the goods of family life that children's right to autonomy looks unenforceable if left to parents. At the same time, the kind of state intervention necessary to 'police' family life is very unattractive: unlikely to succeed, and moreover, threatening to produce great harm that would undermine the essence of family life. Weinstock's solution is to argue that it is not just the family that is responsible for developing children's capacities for autonomous decision-making. The problem of children's autonomy is best thought of, not as a matter of family ethics, but public policy. Political philosophers should thus, in their focus on the politics of childrearing, consider ways in which the obligation to inculcate autonomy resides with state institutions, in particular, the public school system.

Sarah Hannan and R.J. Leland's paper examines yet another entirely different – and in some ways more fundamental – question, which *Family Values* does not directly explore, namely, whether adults' interest in parenting supports a right to procreate. Hannan and Leland argue that although the interest that adults have in engaging in a parent–child relationship may generate a right to parent, as Brighouse and Swift persuasively argue, it does not also support a right for adults to create a child for them to raise. The authors' core and very original argument is that the interest in parenting is essentially tied to what they call the 'bads of childhood'. Childhood, in their view, involves at least four bad conditions: an impaired capacity for practical reasoning, a need for extensive adults' (and especially parental) control, a deep vulnerability, and a lack of stable practical identity. These bads are crucial to explaining the special value of parent-child relationships, according to Hannan and Leland. Adults would not have a special interest in engaging in such relationships if childhood did not have those bad features. So, adults' interest in caring for a child is fundamentally attached to what's bad about being a child. In Hannan and Leland's view, this implies that the interest in parenting cannot support a right for adults to create the need for care by bringing a child into existence.

Harry Brighouse and Adam Swift are the authors of the final paper in the volume, which provides responses to each contribution. Brighouse and Swift express appreciation for all the contributions, endorsing some points, while refining or rejecting others. Certainly the range of stimulating responses to their book is an indication of its significance and interest, as well as the remarkable achievement of its scholarship. Inspired by the feminist critique of the family, political philosophers have only relatively recently looked into questions of justice, equality and autonomy in connection with the relations between parents and children. *Family Values* is an outstanding contribution to the philosophical inquiry as to how personal attachments and political principles may be reconciled. We hope that readers agree that the following collection of excellent essays is a worthy tribute to this important work.

What abolishing the family would not do

Anca Gheaus

ABSTRACT
Because families disrupt fair patterns of distribution and, in particular, equality of opportunity, egalitarians believe that the institution of the family needs to be defended at the bar of justice. In their recent book, Harry Brighouse and Adam Swift have argued that the moral gains of preserving the family outweigh its moral costs. Yet, I claim that the egalitarian case for abolishing the family has been overstated due to a failure to consider how alternatives to the family would also disturb fair distributions and, in particular, equality of opportunity. Absent the family, children would continue to be exposed to care-givers of different levels of ability, investment in childrearing and beneficial partiality. In addition, social mechanisms other than the family would lead to the accumulation of economic inequalities. *Any* kind of upbringing will fail to realise equality for reasons that go deeper than the family: our partiality and unequal abilities to nurture.

Introduction

There is an influential tradition of philosophers worrying that the institution of the family poses a challenge to distributive justice – most importantly (and most unavoidably) to the ideal of equality of opportunity. Following Harry Brighouse and Adam Swift's discussion of this problem in their book *Family Values: The Ethics of Parent-Child Relationships* (2014), I call it 'the egalitarian challenge to the family'. By 'family' one should understand here the raising of children by a very small number of adults, who freely associate with each other and undertake long-term fiduciary responsibilities towards their biological, or adopted, children.

Brighouse and Swift think that taking seriously the egalitarian challenge requires us to ask the question of 'why it would be a bad idea to abolish the family' (2014, p. 4). Their analysis seems to rely on the assumption that, absent the family and other things being equal, there would be significantly less disruption of distributive justice. Yet, such an assumption is too quick. In this paper I question it, and suggest – somewhat speculatively – that the real root of the problem is not the family. Rather, the root of those disruptions of equality the vehicle of which is, in existing societies, the family, is the combination of human partiality and our unequal interest in, and abilities to, nurture others – in particular, children. Since children's (even minimal) development depends on the nurturing they receive from some adults in the context of personal relationships, and since it is not possible to have all children raised by the same person, any upbringing will embody an element of brute luck for children when it comes to the quality of care they receive. The main claim of the paper is that any form of upbringing alternative to the family – whether or not designed with the aim of meeting children's needs as much as it is possible outside the family – will disturb equality, in particular equality of opportunity. Moreover, I raise doubts that equality of opportunity would be any more attainable in a society that rears its children outside the family – that is, in a society without families – than it is in a society with families properly reformed, along egalitarian lines.

This paper is grounded in the belief that partiality is universal, and likely to make its equality-disturbing appearance in any kind of upbringing. Partiality is probably impossible to eradicate and, moreover, desirable. Bernard Williams (1973) thought that one's integrity as an agent depends on allowing one's partial concerns to play an important role in guiding one's action. In other words, agency itself – and, with it, morality – may depend on permitting partiality. I think he was right; and in due course I shall elaborate on the thought that, as children, we need to experience partiality in the form of love if we are to flourish.

My argument, if correct, in no way distracts from the value of considering which *kinds* of family are legitimate given their impact on distributive justice – which is the real aim of Brighouse and Swift's enterprise. But it does bear on the usefulness of framing the discussion in terms of 'abolishing the family' rather than merely reforming it. This is because talk of abolishing the family for the sake of equality may be a red herring (Macleod, 2017): In order to answer the question of whether one has any reason to abolish the family in light of the egalitarian challenge – and even in order to judge whether it is worth engaging with this question – one needs to know if alternative childrearing institutions would be significantly less likely to disrupt fair distributions than a (properly reformed) family. If they would not, then inequalities of opportunity between children raised by different parents cannot, even *prima facie*, be a good reason to abolish the family. Furthermore, talk of abolishing the family also risks to unnecessarily polarise the discussion and antagonise the public – including the academic, and, perhaps, even some of the philosophical, public – which is likely to be detrimental to much needed egalitarian reforms.

The family and patterns of distributions – a brief overview

The ideal of equal opportunity has been interpreted in very different ways, ranging from the belief that there should be a level playing field when it comes to social competition for desirable goods to the thought that we should all have the same chance to be well off, as long as we display the same level of responsible behaviour (Mason, 2006). The family seems to prevent the full realisation of the principle of equal opportunity across the entire range of its possible interpretations. One's family largely determines one's access to a variety of resources that shape one's opportunities: people get jobs based on family relationships – like managing a family business – and have access to privileged sources of information and social connections that tilt the playing field in their favour. Parents shape children's future opportunities by influencing the cultivation of their talents and ambitions. Some parents buy private schooling for their children or use their superior knowledge to send them to better state schools, or they organise additional educational activities (like special holidays and trips to the museum). Micro-interactions between parents and children – such as dinner conversations and the reading of bedtime stories – directly shape children's values, abilities and aspirations. Last, but not least, different children have parents who are unequally good at bringing them up, which results in different opportunities to lead good lives as children and to develop into happy, resourceful and resilient adults.

John Rawls noted that 'the principle of fair opportunity can be only imperfectly carried out, at least as long as the institution of the family exists' (Rawls, 1971, p. 74). He thought that the existence of the family was inconsistent with the full realisation of the just society in which native talent and ambition alone determine individuals' opportunity for socially desirable positions. Yet, parents' level of income and education unavoidably influences the development of their children's talent, and therefore also the opportunities that their children will have, over time, to access wealth, income and positions of power and prestige. These inequalities cannot be justified, on Rawlsian terms, since they are not necessary in order to make the situation of the worst-off members of society as good as possible. Rawls has explicitly wondered, perhaps rhetorically: 'Is the family to be abolished, then?' and gave his own, negative, reasoned answer.

Not only Rawlsians, but also luck egalitarians should be bothered by the impact of the family on just distributions. James Fishkin (1983, p. 3) noted that three principles of justice that are widely endorsed by liberal egalitarians generate a trilemma. These principles demand that social positions be assigned on merit, that individuals enjoy equality of life chances, and that we respect the autonomy of the family. The last of these principles protects parents' freedom to rear their children as they judge fit (within the usual constraints imposed by morality). Yet, for the reasons mentioned above, parental freedom unavoidably translates into unequal life chances for children insofar as desirable resources

– good jobs for instance – are distributed in a competitive manner and according to merit.

But the influence of the family on life chances is not limited to people's access to good jobs, positions of power or social prestige, nor – more generally – to goods whose distribution can, or should, be governed by competition. Egalitarians ought to be concerned about the family, and about childrearing in general, while embracing any of a very wide range of assumptions about what goods, material or not, represent advantage, and how they are to be distributed (competitively or not). For instance, coming to value certain things may itself be a form of advantage, which has a non-competitive, as well as a competitive, dimension – since we could all have worthwhile conceptions of the good. As Veronique Munoz-Dared notes (1999, pp. 40–41), the influence of the family goes beyond its influence on economic or social success, shaping who people are[1] and how they think about a good life:

> as long as there are families, and hence deep inequalities between people's initial circumstances as regard class, social condition, cultivated attitudes to effort, to self-sacrifice, to autonomy, and so on, the ideal of equal realization of people's natural capacities and moral powers, *including their capability to form, revise and pursue their own conception of the good*, shall not be delivered. [my emphasis]

Familial relationship goods as the justification of the family

So, given that the family shapes who we are and how we think about a good life as well as our chances to access this good, what, if anything, can justify it? *Family Values* offers an elaborate argument drawing on the value of parent–child intimacy to explain why, on the balance of reasons, we ought to preserve the family (in a reformed version), in spite of its unavoidable disruption of fairness. This is my own attempt to reconstruct their argument:

(1) The family inevitably disrupts just distributions – and as is, it perpetuates and exacerbates objectionable inequalities of income, status and various other non-material goods; even well regulated, it would undermine equality of opportunity.

(2) But the family is uniquely able to generate, via the parent–child intimacy, very important goods for both children and adults.

(3) The value indicated in (2) is more important than the disvalue indicated in (1).

(4) Therefore, all things considered, reasons of equality of opportunity do not show that the family is morally unjustified.

Many people are convinced that some interpretation of the second premise is correct (Archard, 2003). Yet, the authors of *Family Values* make the strongest case that I know of for this belief, by elaborating on the kinds of goods available only within (good) families, which they call 'familial relationship goods'. They also provide some support for the third premise and, *mutatis mutandis*, for the conclusion. In a nutshell the argument of the book is that the family provides both children and parents – who stand in an authoritative and intimate relationship with children – the good of meeting children's interests in a happy childhood and in physical, emotional, intellectual and social development; the good of giving children and parents a sense of continuity with the past and the future; and, for adults, the good of playing well the parental role. Of these, the most important consideration is the meeting of children's interests. Proper care for children requires the continuity in care uniquely afforded by growing up in a family. On Brighouse and Swift's view, familial relationship goods are very weighty and cannot be substituted by other relationship goods, which makes them a part of the *distribuenda* of justice. Abolishing the family would deprive all individuals – *qua* children and then *qua* adults – of goods to which they ought to have an opportunity.

This defence of the family is not meant to justify anything like the prerogatives that parents currently enjoy with respect to conferring advantage on to their children. Brighouse and Swift note that parents' freedom, for instance, to buy private education, or to bequest large amounts of wealth, cannot be justified by appeal to familial relationship goods. They also advocate egalitarian reforms to ensure that all children, and all adults who wish to parent and can parent well, are able to enjoy familial relationship goods. As I shall explain shortly, Brighouse and Swift do not believe that these reforms can write out *all* inequality of opportunity resulting from different children growing up in different families. But they argue, convincingly, that a world with perfect equality of opportunity yet devoid of the goods of parenting is worse than a world of families and imperfect equality of opportunity.

Indeed, Brighouse and Swift are not the first egalitarians to argue that the egalitarian challenge to the family can be addressed through a radical reform of the family, but they are more explicit than others that no amount of desirable reform can eliminate all inequality of opportunity resulting from childrearing in the family. Others thought that Fishkin's trilemma can be dissolved by rejecting a strong version of the autonomy of the family principle. Peter Vallentyne and Morry Lipson (1989) make this case, noting that today's children will have the right to equal opportunities to pursue their conception of the good once they become adults, and hence today's adults ought to ensure that all children have an equal opportunity to develop the skills they will need for this pursuit. They argue we ought to abandon the principle that protects the current extent of parental freedom and, moreover, to engage in reforms such as the banning of certain adults from parenting, as well as providing state-funded training and information programmes for would-be parents and numerous subsidised educational programmes for children. Such reforms could indeed reduce the inequalities of opportunity between children raised in different families.

But there are good reasons to think, *contra* Vallentyne and Lipson, that even the properly reformed family will remain incompatible with equal opportunities for all to pursue their conception of the good. Assume 100% inheritance taxes, no private education and all the reforms suggested by Vallentyne and Lipson. These measures would fall short of ensuring equally good childhoods to all children and equally favourable conditions for the development of their abilities and values. This is because, as Brighouse and Swift (2014) and Swift in earlier work (2003) noted – drawing on much sociological data – parental influence on children is *to a large extent* exercised through everyday micro-interactions that constitute the very substance of parent–child intimacy, such as the reading of bedtime stories and conversations over dinner. Moreover, as feminists working on the ethics of care have observed, the quality of care that children receive is constitutive of better or worse conditions for them to develop their abilities and conception of the good, including, for instance, a capacity to engage in, sustain and value caring relationships as adults (Gheaus, 2009). Yet, it is most likely impossible to fully monitor and shape parent–child interactions – and even trying to do so would undermine the nurturing intimacy that justifies the family in the first place. So attempts to equalise the effects of family life on children's opportunities are likely to result in the much-dreaded phenomenon of levelling down (Brighouse & Swift, 2014). Further, if micro-interactions are largely responsible for the transmission of advantage, this is probably to be explained, in part, through the fact that different parents have different levels of nurturing ability, views about good parenting and investment in their children. Some are more patient, attentive, affectionate, wise or loving, or willing to dedicate themselves to childrearing than others. Short of assuming that we could equalise people's parenting abilities and investment in parenting, it is difficult to see how the reformed family could prevent inequalities in childrearing. So even the well-reformed family will remain, to some extent, incompatible with equality of opportunity unless all prospective parents become equally competent and invested in their children.

Moreover, Brighouse and Swift's defence of the family is vulnerable to the following worry: even if the family *can* uniquely promote the goods generated by parent–child intimacy, we know it does not *always* do so – that is, it does not generate familial relationships goods for all children. Some children grow up without parents or have parents unable or unwilling to sustain the intimate relationships that Brighouse and Swift deem valuable. They are the 'worst off' when it comes to the goods of family life, and the defence of the family proposed by Brighouse and Swift is irrelevant to them: To these children, the inequalities generated even by a reformed family cannot be justified by appeal to the superior value of familial relationship goods, since these children do not get to enjoy such goods.

Brighouse and Swift may answer this last objection by stressing that they do not defend the family as it is, but as it should be: effective in securing adequate parents to all children. Yet, bringing about such a transformation seems particularly hard because it would require not merely institutional change, but a profound transformation of people's personalities and of their everyday interactions with each other. The elimination of private schooling and inheritance may be politically difficult to achieve, but relatively easy to implement as long as there is a will – unlike the tackling of individuals' unequal ability and willingness to nurture children. It is likely that serious cases of child neglect and abuse can be drastically reduced, although probably not eliminated. But ensuring that all parents are adequate, let alone equally able to provide familial relationship goods, looks like a utopian ideal of a different order.

The case for keeping the family in the face of the egalitarian challenge may therefore seem to depend on whether it is possible to ensure that all children have adequate parents. Before such a radical reform takes place, the inequalities of opportunities faced by children raised in different families remain unjustifiable to those children who are themselves negatively affected without the redeeming enjoyment of any familial relationship goods. Unless, as I explain below, the same inequalities would persist in the absence of the family: in that case the worst off of the family life could be told, by way of justification, that different childrearing practices would generate similar inequalities.

To sum up, even reformed, the family poses a complex egalitarian challenge: First, it continues to disturb equality of opportunity. Second, unless and until all children have adequate parents, it is hard to justify it to those children who are both raised by inadequate parents and are at the losing end of inequalities of opportunities caused by the family. Brighouse and Swift address only the first part of the challenge, and their answer concedes that equality of opportunity is inevitably the loser given the value of family relationships. Showing that equality of opportunity would be similarly disturbed in the absence of the family can also start to answer the second part.

Egalitarian challenges to institutional childrearing

The family is not the source but merely a contingent vehicle of many inequalities of opportunities, whose deepest source lies with human partiality and adults' unequal abilities to nurture children. Moreover, even the current, unreformed, family is merely one of several such vehicles; in its absence, other institutions may promote more partiality-generated inequality then they do now.

I discuss three reasons that jointly suggest that, in the absence of the family, childrearing arrangements will inevitably continue to generate morally objectionable inequalities.[2] They apply, albeit differently, to both adequate and inadequate institutional childrearing arrangements. These reasons are: the fact that different people who raise children will be differently capable to nurture them; the fact that different children will likely enjoy different levels of partiality from their childrearers, that is, some children will be liked and loved more than others;

and the fact that people will, over their lifetime, tend to prefer certain individuals for associative purposes, thus allowing inequalities to cluster over time. Thus, even if material and cultural gifts were to be banned from institutional childrearing (to an extent to which they either cannot or ought not to be banned from the family), material transfers could happen between some childrearers and their grown-up former charges. In addition, depriving people from an opportunity to rear children is likely to channel their partiality towards other individuals.

Differently able and motivated childrearers

Consider a world in which children are being reared in institutions rather than in families. You may imagine these institutions to be akin to permanent boarding schools, in which children are brought up by specialised employees – henceforth 'childrearers'. This is not the only alternative to the family. As Brighouse and Swift note, other possible ways of bringing up children include 'Kibbutzim, in which child raising is shared between "parents" and designated child-raising specialists' and '[c]ommunes in which a large group of adults collectively and jointly raises a group of children, with no adult thinking of herself as having any special responsibility for any particular child, and no child thinking of herself as the responsibility of any particular adult' (Brighouse & Swift, 2014, pp. 70–71). Yet, I assume that state-run institutional childrearing is the most likely setting of fully egalitarian childrearing, and so it provides the best test case for the point I make here.

Munoz-Darde is one of the few philosophers who engage in a systematic exercise of imagining what it would mean to abolish the family and rear children in something akin to 'a very well-run orphanage'. Comparing the family to institutional childrearing, she notes that '[t]he distinctive feature of a society in which children are raised in families is ... that children are looked after by different groups of elders, with different criteria and resources in each instance' (1999, pp. 44–45). By resources here she means material resources. Note that the last two features – different criteria and different material resources – characterise families as we have them now, but they are not crucial for the existence of the family. If we only lived in societies that were egalitarian, in both ethos and material distributions, it would be possible for children to grow up in families that would not disturb equality through differential levels of parental wealth. Sufficient socialisation of children outside the family and public discussion about good childrearing could perhaps generate (compliance with) general criteria of what constitutes good childrearing. Also, if children spent enough time in non-sectarian childrearing institutions they could have access to a variety of values and possible life choices. As for the last feature of the family identified by Munoz-Darde – that different elders rear different children – it is not in fact unique to the family. It would characterise institutional childrearing too, and this fact may be enough to create significant discrepancy in life opportunities.

As already noted, much difference in upbringing may derive from the fact that different children are reared by different individuals with different aptitudes and willingness to invest themselves in childrearing. This means that childrearing outside the family may be just as disturbing of equality of opportunity as a properly reformed family.

I assume – importantly, if somewhat self-evidently – that, in order to qualify as childrearing, any arrangement must enable children to survive and grow up into minimally functional social beings. Some of children's most basic needs are for physical and regular interaction with other people and emotional and intellectual engagement with care-givers. For this reason, any childrearing will rely on some hands-on work done by people (rather than robots).[3] We know that babies whose needs for shelter, food and clothing are met by people, though only mechanically, and are never given any physical affection, emotional care and intellectual stimulation, will suffer from very high morbidity and mortality, fail to develop adequately and often find it impossible to socialise.[4] This means that any upbringing that is humane and socially sustainable will require at least *some* personalised interaction between children and childrearers. Childrearing, however, that serves children's interests better, will go beyond this standard, allowing for plenty of interaction between children and childrearers and encouraging the formation of deep personal bonds.

Further, I assume that childrearers will differ from each other with respect to how well they are able to nurture children. It may be easier to select out abusive or neglectful childrearers than it is to prevent abusive or neglectful parents from raising children. Therefore, by eliminating or significantly reducing neglect and abuse, it may be possible to ensure more equality between children brought up in institutions than we can ensure between children raised in a (reformed) family: the difference between the best and the worst childrearers might be smaller than that between the best and the worst parents. But significant differences would nevertheless exist: amongst non-abusive or neglectful childrearers, and even amongst good childrearers, there is much variation in numerous skills that make children's lives go well and shape their future chances, like attentiveness, patience, mindfulness, kindness or an ability to take pleasure in children.

All these differences will shape children's opportunities in any institutional setting. In institutions designed with the modest aim of allowing children to survive and grow up, but with little interest for the quality of care beyond this standard, the differences between the best and the worst childrearers will likely be larger. Some, but not all, children will be lucky to have decent, or even adequate, childrearers. In institutions designed to advance all children's legitimate interests, childrearers will be, on average, much better, and the differences between them smaller; but allowing children to spend more time in personalised interaction with their childrearers and to form deeper relationships with them will amplify the effect of existing differences. Some of the personal qualities of people who raise us make a significant difference to our quality of life and to our present and future opportunities. Abolishing the family would not eliminate this source of unfairness.

Note that, if it were possible, through training, to turn people into adequate childrearers and therefore diminish some inequalities in upbringing, then this would advance equality independently of the issue of the existence of the family[5]; therefore, if we could eliminate the inequalities stemming from unequal abilities to care in childrearing institutions, we could also do it within the family. Yet, more likely, *any* childrearing arrangement – familial or not, and adequate or not – will end up exposing children to differently resourceful and dedicated adults.

Unequal affection

The second reason to doubt that the abolition of the family could result in an upbringing fully compatible with equality (of opportunity) also has to do with the nature of intimate interactions between children and childrearers. It is very likely that, as long as people – rather than robots – raise children in ways that rely on personalised interaction – rather than on the mechanical carrying out of tasks – some childrearers would get to appreciate the individuality of some children, and become emotionally attached to them (as well as children to childrearers). It is plausible that, unlike the minimally acceptable childrearing, adequate childrearing involves a significant measure of personalised relationships between children and their childrearers. This is in part for epistemic reasons – adequate childrearers are the advocates of children's interests and, therefore, need to know them well.[6] And, in part, it is because only within personalised relationships is it possible to meet children's need to be loved and appraised – both of which require that children feel understood in their individuality. Adequate institutional upbringing would give children this – although, presumably, to a lesser extent than good families and without the important benefits of continuity in care and higher intimacy afforded by family life.

The worry that children raised in institutions could not be loved or liked for their own individuality is often invoked as a main argument for preserving the family (its inegalitarian effects notwithstanding). Without endorsing this worry, Munoz-Darde (1998, pp. 47–8) expresses it well:

> in most cases children in families are treated as ends in themselves, they are cared for as the special person they are, intimate relationships and the language of affection connected with it constituting a force of individuation ... The thought would be that children need to be treated partially, as the singular person they are, in order to flourish. ... how probable is that, were the family to entirely disappear? Would not my fantasy of a generalized boarding school with teachers devoted to the individuality of each child vanish, were the state to have the sole control of the upbringing of children? Wouldn't it be the case that children would then be brought up not as ends in themselves, but as mere means for a collective purpose?

Here, our imagination may be unduly dominated by the bleak representations of orphanages in the collective imaginary – institutions where cold, detached adults perform, mechanically, a restrictive set of duties. However, note that even Dickens-inspired orphanages would most likely generate inequality of opportunity since every now and then a child would be lucky to be raised by an affectionate childrearer; the difference in quality of life and future prospects between such a child and the rest would be huge. No orphanage in which children are able to survive could realise levelling down in this respect.

But there is of course no reason to think that a 'well-run orphanage' would display this feature, nor is it unimaginable that children be raised in an institutional setting where their carers are humane and numerous enough to pay proper attention to their charges. Munoz-Darde probably echoes a general worry when she writes that, without the family, people would not 'have the special ties of sentiment that in families parents often have towards their offspring'.[7] In a similar spirit, Brighouse and Swift note that the family is the 'natural home of affectionate relationships' (Brighouse & Swift, 2014, p. 4). The worry may be warranted in a strong interpretation – possibly, without the family, children and childrearers would tend not to forge emotional relationships that are quite as deep and enduring as those between parents and children. But there is no reason to think that they would not forge nurturing emotional relationships at all. Why wouldn't they? Many people think that the biological connection between parents and children guarantees the 'special' nature of the parent–child sentimental ties – in which case upbringing outside the biological family could not, in general, produce them (Brighouse and Swift do not seem to endorse this belief). Even if this was the case, sufficient ties of sentiment could be forged in childrearing institutions to allow some loving relationships between children and childrearers. To many people – presumably even more so to those who would choose to work as childrearers – children are particularly lovable individuals, and we know that non-biological parents can and do love their children. And, if the family did not exist, other settings would become the natural home of relationships based on love.

But if children and childrearers would be sufficiently close to each other to meet children's needs, then it is very likely that childrearers would tend to like and love the children in their charge differently. Loving parents, after all, are often known to like and even love some of their children more than others. This, at least, is what we know from anecdotal evidence and fiction, although it is probably a difficult fact for parents to admit. Some will worry that a parent who likes or loves one of her children more than others – or at least who lets this show – is, for this reason, not an adequate parent. It is an interesting question whether it would be, all-things-considered, desirable if childrearers raising children in institutions were always impartial towards their charges. Demanding impartiality from childrearers, and subjecting children to impartial upbringing, might in fact be undesirable for all parties.

But, desirable or not, it would in any case be unrealistic to assume that people engaged in long-term caring relationships can remain impartial towards those they are caring for. (This may be unrealistic even in the case of fiduciary relationships that are more episodic in nature, such as teaching and doctoring.) Just as we have no reason to assume that institutional childrearing will necessarily select the coldest, most emotionally detached of people, we have no reason to think that childrearers will be so different, morally speaking, from the rest of us so as to be able to always be impartial. Yet, if how much we are – and know we are – liked or loved as children makes a significant difference to how well our lives go, including to our future opportunities, we have another reason to think that upbringing outside the family will continue to generate morally arbitrary inequality.

It is not parents' or childrearers' partiality as such that (keeping equal other things such as ability to confer advantage) translates into more inequalities in upbringing, but differences between the level of partiality that different parents or childrearers display. I do not see a reason to think that the partiality gap between the more partial and the less partial parents is wider than the partiality gap between the more partial and the less partial childrearers. One may think that an advantage of institutional childrearing – especially of the adequate kind – is that it assigns more than two childrearers to each child, thereby increasing every child's chances to be cared for by someone who gives the child loving affection.[8] But this attractive feature can be secured while preserving the family, by introducing mandatory substantial non-parental care from an early age – a reform which, as I argued elsewhere, we have many reasons to support (Gheaus, 2011).

Now, it is possible that universal, adequate, legitimate and sustainable institutional childrearing is not possible, at least by liberal lights. Adequate childrearing may require continuity in childcare, which in turn seems incompatible with occupational freedom for childrearers. And universal institutional childrearing may result, over time, in state-enforced similarity, robbing individuals of their chance to experiment with different values and life style – at least, this is Munoz-Darde's and, possibly, Rawls's worry. Maybe it would also rob children of adequate attention and love from adults. These consequences would depend on how resilient love and diversity really are. Even more plausible, and relevant to the purpose of this discussion, is that universal institutional childrearing might not be able to serve children's interests *better* than the family does (especially a properly reformed family.) However, this is not a challenge to the argument I offer here: *in*adequate childrearing institutions, we have seen, also display the above discussed sources of inequality between children. Even more than in adequate institutions, inadequate institutions would have children raised by differently able and motivated childrearers; and some children would be loved (I assume that love is at least that resilient!), while others would not.

If any reasonably imaginable upbringing would expose children to people with unequal childrearing abilities and to unequal levels of affection, it is very likely that the family is merely a contingent vehicle of inequalities stemming from childrearing. In the absence of the family, other vehicles of generating unfair inequalities via human partiality, including institutional childrearing, would probably be more effective than they can be in a world of families.

The Catholic Church (or something like it)

Finally, it is a commonplace that the family also contributes to the intergenerational transmission of inequalities by allowing related individuals to accumulate, over time, large amounts of wealth. Since being well-off most often facilitates, and sometimes is a requirement for, being able to accumulate even more wealth, families allow wealth to cluster over time. What is true of wealth often applies to other desirable goods, such as valuable career opportunities or opportunities for personal development. Frequently, families are associations of individuals who are equally well or equally poorly connected to other well (or poorly) connected and educated people. Yet, the family is not unique in this respect. The Catholic Church is an example of how partiality between people who have no family relationships can similarly disrupt equality of opportunities. A just society would not allow an accumulation of intergenerational wealth similar to that of the Catholic Church, but it will probably nevertheless allow people to associate in (intergenerational) associations which inevitably distribute opportunities very unequally.

Now, assume that in a society that lacks the family, and that is otherwise just, people are permitted to accumulate wealth over their life time, associate freely with others, make gifts and benefit others by providing them with valuable social relations. And imagine that children were all raised in adequate institutions, giving them as-equal-as-possible – in light of the above-discussed constraints – starts in the competition for social goods, by providing them with the same quality of schooling and extra-curricular activities. Depending on how competitive the distribution of goods would be in that society (which surely is a matter of justice independent from that of the existence of the family), individuals would be able to accumulate more or less wealth over the course of their life.

Since, throughout their lives, people would be free to associate with others, it is likely that they would form associations based in part on acquaintance and personal similarities – just as people do in existing societies. Sometimes caregivers and their now adult former charges would (continue to) be friends. And often the more enterprising, popular, skilled and motivated individuals would likely benefit from each others' support and thus enjoy increasingly better opportunities.

Most importantly, individuals would probably want to use the wealth they accumulate in order to advance some of their personal goals. Throughout their lives, and especially towards the end of their lives, accumulated wealth could turn into substantial gifts for those they love or for organisations and causes they support. Redistributive mechanisms will presumably regulate the extent to which free association can impact on equality of opportunity (and this is an issue orthogonal to that of the existence of the family). But, if partiality is both desirable and unavoidable – as I assume it is – redistributive mechanisms will not operate by trying to eliminate free association itself; any plausible conception of the exercise of legitimate political power must ensure that individuals have some space for personal relationships and some freedom to benefit those about whom they care most. In existing societies, most individuals care predominantly about the well-being of their children. But, not having children 'of their own', people living in societies without families would most likely be a lot more invested in their friendships than are people who raise families. In all likelihood, even in a society displaying an egalitarian ethos, personal relationship would, and should, continue to matter to people as much as they matter now. With parenting unavailable, other relationships would take the central stage. Hence, people would gift and bequest wealth to their friends, sometimes younger ones. In this way, inequality could be perpetuated – and accumulated – across generations even in the absence of the family, thanks to the same partiality that perpetuates inequalities via familial relationships in the world as we know it.

In addition, because they could not raise children, people would probably channel more interests into various institutions meant to serve various causes. These institutions would become another important mechanism for the intergenerational reproduction of inequality. Even in a world of families, there are associational institutions other than the family that contribute significantly to the intergenerational reproduction of inequality – including inequality of opportunity. As mentioned, an example of such existing institution – which, interestingly, functions for many people (priests, nuns and monks) as an *alternative* to the family – is the Catholic Church. Through an accumulation of gifts and the pooling of non-material resources over time, this institution has achieved a massive accumulation of wealth and power and therefore undermined equality of opportunity. (And even in just societies a similar development would have been likely, albeit on a different scale.) Absent the family, associational institutions that capture individuals' allegiances – religious, like churches, but also non-religious, like clubs – would probably become even more significant vehicles of inequality of opportunities than they are now.

Of course, it may be that in a just world there would be equality-justified restrictions on how much wealth one can accumulate over a lifetime, on associational practices including professional networking, on gifts and bequests and on the scope of social competition for various goods. But, again, in this case – in a world of, say, functional socialism or communism – it is not clear that the family would really have more potential for disrupting equality than other permitted private associations that, in the absence of the family, could take a more central role in people's lives.

This is not to say that abolishing the family now, in the world as we have it, and rearing children in well-run, egalitarian institutions, would not boost equality. But the boost would be due to the dismantling of large fortunes and social capital accumulated over generations, and not to eliminating the features that make the family unavoidably equality-disrupting. This means that a similar boost of equality could be achieved without abolishing the family – simply by allowing public institutions to take over the education and socialisation of children to a significant extent, while at the same time implementing the usual economic measures advocated by egalitarians. It may be the case that abolishing the family is the most efficient *shortcut* to a more egalitarian world. But, if I am right, a world without the family will likely fall significantly short of full equality of opportunity, while a world with the family can get us as close to equality of opportunity as it is possible given human partiality and differences in nurturing abilities.

Conclusion

I have argued that human partiality and unequal abilities to nurture would likely disrupt equality (of opportunity) in any imaginable form of bringing up children – and, in particular in one that we can expect to meet, even minimally, children's current and developmental needs. Whatever else it could accomplish, the abolition of the family would not allow for the realisation of equality (of opportunity) since it is not the source of inequality.

If so, it is not obvious that what Brighouse and Swift (and many others) consider to be an egalitarian challenge to the family really is a challenge to the *family*. More likely, the challenge is to human partiality and unequal nurturing abilities. And, for better or worse, we are not likely to be able to change these facts. In this case, it seems misleading to frame the discussion of the much-needed egalitarian reform of the family in terms of questioning its very existence. The defence proposed by Brighouse and Swift – that familial relationship goods are more important than equality of opportunity – may not be convincing to the worst-off of the family. But if a world of perfect equality of opportunity is not possible, it is not clear that the family's disruption of equality of opportunity is a reason for abolishing it – even a *prima facie* one. The matter depends on whether institutional childrearing would, in fact, disturb equality of opportunity significantly less than the (properly reformed) family. It is this last claim that my paper puts into question.

Notes

1. She writes that the family affects 'not only our opportunities in life, but the kind of person we become'. While she is not herself insisting on this point, this includes matters of character and personality.
2. Perhaps inequalities with respect to some goods – such as worthwhile conceptions of the good – would not be quite as large as they are in the absence of the family; but inequalities of wealth and income, that are most usually discussed by philosophers of the family, possibly would.
3. The same assumptions about children's needs are made by Brighouse and Swift.
4. This is indicated by longitudinal studies on children growing up in Romanian orphanages (Nelson, Fox, & Zeanah, 2014; Zeanah, Smyke, Koga, Carlson, & The Bucharest Early Intervention Project Core Group, 2005). Of course, the children in these studies often suffered various forms of abuse alongside emotional neglect. But other studies on institutional childrearing show that emotional neglect *in itself* has very detrimental effects (The St. Petersburg—USA Orphanage Research Team, 2009).
5. Trainings for parents – both to prepare them to enter parenthood and to help them get better while at it – is also one of the measures proposed by Vallentyne and Lipson.
6. For an account of the instrumental value of parents having close knowledge of their children, see Anne Alstott (2004). Since these reasons have to do with child well-being, her point applies to the imaginary childrearers, although they would not have the same opportunities to know the children in their charge as parents would.
7. Worry which she does not necessarily endorse herself (Munoz-Darde, 1998, p. 44).
8. I am grateful to an anonymous referee for alerting me to this possibility.

Acknowledgements

For comments and suggestions I am grateful to David Archard, Andrée-Anne Cormier, Serena Olsaretti, Liam Shields, Adam Swift, Christine Sypnowich and an anonymous referee of CRISPP.

Disclosure statement

No potential conflict of interest was reported by the author.

Funding

This project has received funding from the European Research Council (ERC) under the European Union's Horizon 2020 Research and Innovation programme [Grant Agreement Number: 648610].

References

Alstott, A. (2004). *No exit: What parents owe society and what society owes parents*. Oxford: Oxford University Press.

Archard, D. (2003). *Children, family and the state*. London: Ashgate.

Brighouse, H., & Swift, A. (2014). *Family values: The ethics of parent-child relationships*. Princeton: Princeton University Press.

Fishkin, J. (1983). *Justice, equal opportunity and the family*. New Haven, CT: Yale University Press.

Gheaus, A. (2009). How much of what matters can we redistribute? love, justice, and luck. *Hypatia, 24*(4), 63–83.

Gheaus, A. (2011). Arguments for nonparental care for children. *Social Theory and Practice, 37*(3), 483–509.

Macleod, C. (2017). Equality and family values: Conflict or harmony? *Critical Review of International and Social Political Philosophy*.

Mason, A. (2006). *Levelling the playing field: The idea of equal opportunity and its place in Egalitarian thought*. Oxford: Oxford University Press.

Munoz-Darde, V. (1998). Rawls, justice in the family and justice of the family. *The Philosophical Quarterly, 48*(192), 335–352.

Munoz-Darde, V. (1999). Is the family to be abolished then? *Proceedings of the Aristotelian Society, 99*(1), 37–56.

Nelson, C. A., Fox, N. A., & Zeanah, C. H. (2014). *Romania's abandoned children: Deprivation, brain development, and the struggle for recovery*. Cambridge, MA: Harvard University Press.

Rawls, J. (1971). *A theory of justice*. Cambridge, MA: Harvard University Press.

Swift, A. (2003). *How not to be a hypocrite: School choice for the morally perplexed parent*. London: Routledge.

The St. Petersburg—USA Orphanage Research Team. (2009). The effects of early social-emotional and relationship experience on the development of young orphanage children. *Monogr Soc Res Child Dev., 73*(3), doi:https://doi.org/10.1111/j.1540-5834.2008.00483.x. Retrieved from http://www.ncbi.nlm.nih.gov/pmc/articles/PMC2702123/pdf/nihms-84380.pdf

Vallentyne, P., & Lipson, M. (1989). Equal opportunity and the family. *Public Affairs Quarterly, 3*(4), 29–47.

Williams, B. (1973). A critique of utilitarianism. In J. J. C. Smart & B. Williams (Eds.), *Utilitarianism: For and against* (pp. 75–150). Cambridge: Cambridge University Press.

Zeanah, C. H., Smyke, A. T., Koga, S. K., Carlson, E., & The Bucharest Early Intervention Project Core Group. (2005). Attachment in institutionalized and community children in Romania. *Child Development, 76*(5), 1015–1028.

Equality and family values: conflict or harmony?

Colin M. Macleod

ABSTRACT
This paper provides a critical commentary on the claim advanced by Harry Brighouse and Adam Swift in their book *Family Values: The Ethics of Parent–Child Relationships* that there is an ineliminable conflict between relationship goods and fair equality of opportunity. I argue there need be no conflict between family values and equality of opportunity in a suitably non-hierarchical society. I also argue that the idea that equality of opportunity might be served by abolishing the family is mistaken. Egalitarian justice does not provide an obstacle to the realization of family values.

Family Values: The Ethics of Parent–Child Relationships[1] is an excellent and important book. It presents a compelling account of the valuable relationship goods made available to children and parents in successful families and explains why access to these goods matters from the point of view of justice. Although they do not emphasize the point, Brighouse and Swift helpfully recognize that the 'relationship goods' that lie at the heart of their conception of family values can be accessed by a wide variety of family types (p. 76). Relationship goods may be accessed not only in 'traditional' families in which married, monogamous, heterosexual couples raise their biological offspring but also in 'non-traditional' families such as those formed by same-sex couples and families with adopted children. The book also illuminates the significance for broadly egalitarian accounts of justice of the recognition of the goods of family. On this matter, two themes of their analysis are particularly interesting. First, Brighouse and Swift argue that there is an *ineliminable* tension between the facilitation of relationship goods in families and even putatively modest egalitarian principles of justice such as fair equality of opportunity. They suggest ways in which this tension can be managed and they deny that parents have strong rights to confer unfair advantages on their children. Nonetheless, they doubt that egalitarian distributive ideals can be fully harmonized with family values and that potentially significant trade-offs between competing values must inevitably be confronted. Second, they argue that given the importance of relationship goods as a source of human flourishing, justice must concern itself with the adequate and fair provision of meaningful opportunities for people to enjoy the goods of family life. There are various ways in which social, political, and material circumstances can be inhospitable to the creation and maintenance of families in which relationship goods can be reliably accessed. Brighouse and Swift correctly point out that the terms on which different people can access and enjoy relationship goods is itself an important matter of justice.

Although neither of these themes is entirely new, Brighouse and Swift explore them in an especially nuanced and careful fashion and thereby advance debate considerably. The richness of their discussion combined with the fact that I find myself in substantive agreement with Brighouse and Swift on so many topics, makes the task of providing a critical commentary on their book especially difficult. To a large degree, the remarks I offer are complementary to the main arguments in the book concerning justice and the family. However, I think there is greater harmony between family values and egalitarian justice than Brighouse and Swift allow. So in what follows, I shall present an analysis of the relation between justice and family values that differs from the position taken by Brighouse and Swift. Whereas Brighouse and Swift treat valuable 'familial relationships as obstacles to the realization of egalitarian ideals' (p. 147), I argue that family values can be facilitated without compromising egalitarian justice. Brighouse and Swift see a competition between important values that calls for an all-things-considered judgment as to how rival values are to be fairly balanced. By contrast, I think that egalitarian ideals do not need to be qualified or limited in order to give recognition to family values. A troubling tension between equality and relationship goods only arises if problematic assumptions about what egalitarianism permits outside the realm of the family are left unchallenged. It is important to emphasize that the difference in our positions is subtle. Thus I agree with Brighouse and Swift when they say: 'the conflict between the family and equality is much less stark than is commonly recognized' (p. 147). But perhaps there is even less conflict than Brighouse and Swift suppose.

Equality of opportunity and relationship goods

Brighouse and Swift devote much of their analysis of justice to discussing the nature and implications of the ideal of fair equality of opportunity. They fall short of actually endorsing fair equality of opportunity as a complete conception of justice but contend that examination of equality of opportunity is worthwhile because it enjoys a certain degree of rhetorical force and popularity in public discourse. Equality of opportunity does not address all facets of justice that are relevant to children and families and thus offers, at best, a partial account of family justice. For instance, because it is oriented to fairness between adults for the pursuit of social positions and employment, it does not address questions about the distribution of resources and opportunities in childhood that have little or no bearing on preparing children for the labor market or citizenship. But since Brighouse and Swift devote a good deal of attention to equality of opportunity in relation to family values, it provides a useful focus of discussion.

The first thing to be observed is that the lip service that is paid to equality of opportunity in contemporary democratic societies seldom grapples with the full implications of the ideal. Consider the familiar characterization of fair equality of opportunity provided by Rawls and cited by Brighouse and Swift (p. 28). Fair equality of opportunity requires: 'not merely that public offices and social positions be open in the formal sense, but that all should have a fair chance to attain them. To specify the idea of a fair chance we say: supposing that there is a distribution of native endowments, those with the same level of talent and ability and the same willingness to use these gifts should have the same prospects of success regardless of their social class of origin' (Rawls, 2001, pp. 43–44). Pursuing equality of opportunity requires reducing and ideally eliminating differences in the social circumstances of children that bear upon the acquisition of the knowledge, skills and dispositions relevant to successful pursuit of employment and social positions.

Brighouse and Swift remind us that, relative to the current circumstances in most liberal democratic states, progress toward realization of equality of opportunity requires radical changes in the structure of political institutions and the distribution of resources and opportunities to people. This is true even if we optimistically assume that formal obstacles to equal opportunity grounded in discrimination on the basis of race, gender, ethnicity and class have been eliminated. Focusing on how families are relevant to achieving the ideal, Brighouse and Swift identify 'the myriad ways in which a child's prospects are influenced by her familial circumstances' (p. 29) and note that 'Children of wealthy parents will have access to high quality schooling, food, health care, housing and holidays, that are bound to foster development in ways not available to children born into poverty' (p. 28). Add to this the way family background affects access to social networks and the acquisition of valuable social capital, the way parents are differentially informed about choices that can help their children compete, and the different degree of engagement parents have in promoting the prospects of their children. Given all these factors, it will seem apparent that the family generates many significant obstacles to equality of opportunity.

So there appears to be a dilemma facing equality of opportunity:

> Fully to realize fair equality of opportunity would require drastic measures. Either we would have to eliminate all the relevant inequalities between parents, in which case we'd need equality of outcome with respect to all things that are helpful to children's development. Or we would have to eliminate all the mechanisms by which inequalities between parents generate unequal developmental

> opportunities for children. Since those mechanisms extend to the very core of the parent-child relationship, the latter seems to imply the abolition of the family as the social institution in which children are raised (p. 30).

Brighouse and Swift are sympathetic to significantly reducing the inequalities between parents of the sort that permit some parents to confer advantages on their children and that thereby disrupt fair equality of opportunity. However, they contend that even if eliminating these inequalities was feasible and attractive, it would not suffice to fully secure fair equality of opportunity. The reason, in effect, is that permitting families to pursue relationship goods inevitably generates unfair inequalities between children.

> The inequalities between children, as far as their developmental opportunities are concerned, stem from processes more central to – one might say constitutive of – family life than egalitarians might have hoped. It seems to be the informal interactions – the bedtime stories, the talk at the table, the family culture, the parenting styles, the inculcation of attitudes and values (some conscious, some unconscious) – that make the difference to children's prospects (pp. 32–33).

As Brighouse and Swift see it, there is a deep tension between family values and egalitarian ideals, albeit one that can be somewhat mitigated both by limiting background inequalities between parents and by limiting some of the ways parents may confer advantages on their children. Nonetheless, they represent the problem as a matter of devising an appropriate *balance* between egalitarian ideals and family values. In this balancing, we must recognize that trade-offs between equality and familial relationship goods are inevitable.

It's important to emphasize that Brighouse and Swift represent the conflict as one that obtains not only in non-ideal circumstances in which there are vast unjust inequalities and the prospects of moving close to fair equality of opportunity are remote.[2] They also contend that the conflict arises at the level of ideal theory. Thus, they think we have reason 'not to pursue fair equality of opportunity all the way' (p. 44) because full realization of the ideal of fair equality of opportunity would 'cost too much in terms of family relationship goods' (p. 44).[3] They insist that the conflict between the family and fair equality of opportunity 'runs deeper than many progressives have wanted to believe' (p. 32). Brighouse and Swift allow that the prerogative of parents to confer some unfair advantages on their children can be circumscribed without jeopardizing relationship goods. However, they think that efforts to completely tame the mechanisms through which parents confer unfair advantages on their children would be antithetical to healthy, intimate relations between parents and children. For example, whereas family relationships can flourish even if parents are prohibited from sending their children to advantage-conferring private schools, valuable relationships between parents and children would be damaged if parents were prevented (somehow) from reading bedtime stories to their children.

Abolishing the family?

I want to consider the underlying diagnosis of the tension between equality and family values. But let me first comment upon the specter of family abolition. The suggestion that full fidelity to egalitarian values might require abolition of the family is noted by Brighouse and Swift as a way of dramatizing the potentially radical and unpalatable implications of adopting an unqualified commitment to egalitarian justice. After describing the informal mechanisms within families that can disrupt equality of opportunity they say: 'This suggests that the only way to deliver fair equality of opportunity would be to get rid of parent-child relationships – to abolish the family – altogether' (p. 33).[4]

However, the concern about the abolition of the family strikes me as a red herring. Abolishing the family as the principal social institution for rearing children would only serve fair equality of opportunity if there is a feasible alternative arrangement that would both better equalize opportunities between children and meet the emotional needs of children at least as well as families. Neither condition is likely to obtain. Consider first that in any large scale, non-family scheme for raising children there will be a division of labor in which different caregivers will inevitably have responsibility for different children. This will be so even if the children are raised by a variety of caregivers. Just as we can expect some variation in the approaches that parents take to rearing children, we can expect variation in the approaches that would be taken by, say, state supplied caregivers in different childrearing centers. The kinds of variation in informal interactions between children and parents that Brighouse and Swift believe upset equality of opportunity when families raise children will almost certainly arise in any non-family arrangement in which children have caregivers and those caregivers differ in their personalities, attitudes and the manner in which they exercise discretion in making a wide variety of child-rearing decisions.

Second, if we allow, as I think we should, that children have a justice-based entitlement to enjoy an ongoing intimate relationship with caregivers who can understand, appreciate, and interact with children who have distinct personalities, cares and challenges, then the provision of an adequate alternative to the family will have to permit, and indeed, foster close emotional bonds between specific children and specific caregivers.[5] Once nurturing children is suitably particularized in a non-family system then it seems doubtful that the equality-disrupting effects of differential parenting can be better avoided in a non-family system for rearing children. The general point here is that talk of abolishing the family only has rhetorical force against pursuing equality of opportunity if one can readily envision an alternative to the family that credibly serves equality of opportunity better than the family can when suitably egalitarian background social and political institutions[6] are in place.

Facilitating relationship goods

In order to realize relationship, goods parents need to have the prerogative to express their care and affection for their children in distinctive ways. They must be able to engage in shared activities with their children and they must be able to manifest concern for the well-being of their children by acting in ways that allow children to have happy and fulfilling childhoods which also cultivate skills, dispositions, and knowledge that can contribute to them leading good lives as adults. It is through acting, in a spontaneous manner that is not encumbered by excessive self-monitoring, on the commitment to care for their own children that parents can confer advantages on their children that disrupt equality of opportunity. Now Brighouse and Swift are careful to deny that parents have a right to confer equality-disrupting advantages on their children. For instance, wealthy parents do not have the right to send their children to elite private schools and a just state may legitimately prevent parents from acting in this way by eliminating or severely circumscribing the degree to which (superior) private education is available for parents to purchase. Blocking the purchase of advantage-conferring private education is acceptable because the achievement of familial intimacy does not depend on being able to benefit one's children in this way. In the normal case, parents who are prevented from sending their children to elite private schools do not thereby lose intimacy with their children. In this sort of case, relationship goods and equality do not compete because valuable expressions of parental affection and concern can be disconnected from the mechanisms that generate problematic inequalities.

However, in a range of other cases it seems much harder to disentangle parental conduct that is integral to the realization of relationship goods from the unfair advantages that the conduct generates. The reading of bedtime stories to children is illustrative of these seemingly more troubling cases. The reading of a bedtime story to a child is a shared, valuable activity that both expresses parental care and affection for children and contributes to the creation and sustenance of an intimate relationship between parents and children. However, the practice of reading stories also contributes to cognitive development and the acquisition of skills and knowledge that have competitive value. So if some parents read to their children and others do not, then fair equality of opportunity can be disrupted: children to whom stories have been read will tend to do better in school than those who did have stories read to them. Differential school performance in turn creates inequalities in the access that otherwise equally talented children have to careers and social positions.

We can view the argument for the *ineliminable* tension between family values and equality of opportunity as resting on four main premises. First, some parental activities or projects integral to the creation and maintenance of highly valuable relationship goods can create competitively valuable skills or other attributes. Call this *skill development*. Second, there are likely to be significant differences between parents both in their abilities to foster skill development in their children and in their interest in engaging in the kinds of family activities that foster skill development. Call this *diverse parenting*. (If all parents were equally well placed and equally inclined to, say, read bedtime stories, then the practice of reading bedtime stories would not disrupt equality of opportunity.) Third, efforts to prevent equality disruption by directly limiting how parents may, in ordinary family contexts, interact with their children would be corrosive to the pursuit of relationship goods. A state policy that sought to closely monitor and tightly regulate everyday interactions between parents and children would be an Orwellian nightmare that would undermine the privacy and spontaneity of interactions between parents and children on which relationship goods depend.[7] Call this *corrosive intervention*. Fourth, institutional structures and policies external to the family cannot mitigate or compensate for the equality disrupting effects arising out of the diversity of parenting styles and their effects on skill development. Call this *ineffective mitigation*.

I readily grant the truth of *corrosive intervention*. So we can set it aside. I also accept that in some contexts *skill development* combined with *diverse parenting* can disrupt fair equality of opportunity. The question is whether this is inevitably so such that we must balance family values against fair equality of opportunity. To frame the discussion, it's worth noting that any tension between relationship goods and equality is a contingent one rather than one that reflects something about the inherent normative structure of relationship goods and equality. It is perfectly conceivable that the differences in the capacities and motivations of parents to engage in skill development could be negligible. For example, all parents could be willing and able to read bedtime stories to their children.

Similarly, to the degree that parenting styles differ, the effects of diverse parenting on skill development could also be negligible. Parents that read to their children might not enhance their children's skills and cognitive development any more than parents who seldom read stories but who frequently play board games with their children. It is plausible to suppose that skill development of the sort relevant to fair equality of opportunity is variously realizable. So diverse parenting does not strictly entail significant differences in skill development between children.

The point here is connected to a more general point about the relation between partiality and equality. Each person can care more about the welfare of specific people to whom they have close affective ties than the welfare of strangers without such partiality colliding with an egalitarian distributive ideal. For instance, people can enjoy both equally good life prospects and close personal friendships characterized by partiality, providing the cumulative effects of partiality on each person's life prospects are roughly the same. The love that my wife and I have for our son might improve his life prospects relative to children who do not benefit from parental love. But loving our son (and not other children) is entirely compatible with other parents loving their children and with other children enjoying equal life prospects.

Of course, the recognition that there is no in principle conflict between relationship goods and equality only partially resolves the putative conflict of values that concerns Brighouse and Swift. They might reasonably contend that the in principle compatibility of values is of little interest if significant conflicts between equality and family values will, in practice, inevitably arise. If this is the case, then we will almost certainly be forced to make an all-things-considered judgment about how to best balance values that conflict in practice. The question is then whether family values and equality can be *realistically* harmonized.

Hierarchy and family values

In considering this question, it helps to distinguish two contexts in which the question can be posed. First, we may consider whether harmonization is realistic in conditions that roughly parallel the current political circumstances in liberal democracies in which there are vast social and economic inequalities and in which competition between people for secure and decently remunerated positions is often fierce. These are conditions in which hierarchies of class are pronounced and in which one's overall life prospects are highly influenced by one's location in the class structure. Second, we may consider the prospects for harmonization in more broadly egalitarian circumstances in which hierarchies of class are much less pronounced and in which one's overall life prospects are not highly determined by one's class position. In this kind of non-hierarchical political community, there would be public provision of universal and uniformly excellent education, health care, day care as well as generous public provision of parks, recreation facilities and community centers. Note that these kinds of institutional arrangements do not regulate the internal life of families and hence are not corrosive to familial relationship goods. (Indeed, they arguably make pursuit of relationship goods easier.) However, they do shape the context in which families exist and arguably influence the incentives that parents have with respect to caring for their children.

Against this background, I want to advance three claims. First, fidelity to fair equality of opportunity plausibly requires establishment of a non-hierarchical political community. Second, in a non-hierarchical political community it is realistic to suppose that equality of opportunity and relationship goods can be harmonized. This is both because the effects of *skill development* and *diverse parenting* will be modest and because well-functioning public institutions can fairly address differences in skill development between children. Third, Brighouse and Swift do not fully appreciate the potential of this route to the harmonization of values because they implicitly expect the dynamics at play in hierarchical political communities that give rise to a tension between equality and family values to obtain in non-hierarchical communities.[8] In effect, they extend claims about *skill development*, *diverse parenting*, and *ineffective mitigation* that are highly plausible in hierarchical political communities to non-hierarchical communities where they are much less plausible.

I will say little about the first claim since it reflects, I think, common ground that Brighouse, Swift and I share. Outside the family, equalizing the opportunity that children have to develop talents and acquire skills surely requires that they have reliable and equal access to good schools and that their capacity to benefit from education is not impaired by poverty, poor health or unpleasant or unsafe living conditions. Taking equality of opportunity seriously involves ensuring that all children have equal access at least to the developmental opportunities that can be provided outside the family. As Brighouse and Swift observe: 'Equality of opportunity is concerned to equalize people's circumstances – in particular, their developmental opportunities' (p. 38). Similarly, if there are huge differences in the overall life prospects that attach to pursuit of different careers and social positions, then the scope for differences in social capital between families of a sort that affect developmental opportunities will be unacceptably wide. So although some differences in remuneration etc. for different careers and social positions are consistent with equality of opportunity, the differences must be such that they do not generate large disparities in social capital between classes. Equalizing developmental opportunities plausibly requires the creation of a largely non-hierarchical political community.

Let's turn to my second claim. We can allow that even in a non-hierarchical political community *skill development* and *diverse parenting* would obtain to some degree. Yet the scope and significance of these factors on the developmental opportunities for children is likely to be modest at best. To begin with, unlike a hierarchical society there would not be vast differences in the capacities or opportunities that parents have to impart useful skills to their children. For example, obstacles that some parents currently face in reading to their children would be radically reduced. Here, it is important to emphasize that the advantages that well-heeled and highly educated parents currently enjoy in conferring advantages on their children are themselves the product of a hierarchical system. And those advantages would be greatly diminished in a non-hierarchical society. The differences in the informal relations between children and parents from different classes that Brighouse and Swift flag as important in influencing children's prospects (p. 127) would diminish as sharp class distinctions themselves were eliminated.

Of course, different parents with different skill sets and different motivations might still impart (whether consciously or not) different skills to their children. But the fact that children acquire different skills from their families need not offend equality of opportunity providing that the skills they do acquire are suitably socially valorized. The child of a musician may acquire more musical training at home than the child of an entrepreneur who gains business acumen from her upbringing. Yet this difference need not yield unfair disparities in children's opportunity sets providing that the life prospects linked to different career paths are reasonably comparable. The opportunity sets of children do not need to be strictly identical in order for them to be relevantly equal.[9]

Finally, to the degree that *skill development* and *diverse parenting* yield some developmental inequalities, the institutions and policies of a non-hierarchical society are well-placed to effectively mitigate them. For example, excellent schools would seek to identify and remedy skill deficits between children and would afford them opportunities to explore and develop talents that parents do not recognize or lack the wherewithal to nurture at home. The fact that some parents cultivate potentially valuable musical, esthetic or physical skills via family activities or projects while others do not would have only a negligible effect on the overall equality of developmental opportunities between children if schools have excellent programs in these domains that are readily accessible by all children. Note finally, that the features and effects of a non-hierarchical society that I have emphasized here are entirely compatible with the flourishing of familial relationship goods. Parents may form close bonds with their children and include them in distinctive activities that are emotionally rewarding. Similarly, the natural concern of parents to promote the well-being of their children can be pursued without meddling interference in the internal lives of the families by the state. Equality of opportunity and family values can be harmonized through a suitable division of moral labor and good institutional design.

The foregoing speculations about the features of a non-hierarchical community may seem like an exercise in utopian political philosophy. After all, we are a long way from creating genuinely non-hierarchical societies and the political prospects for radical transformation of existing communities are currently rather bleak. Nonetheless, I think the position I have sketched is 'realistically utopian' (Rawls, 2001, p. 4). The imagined community does not violate the strains of commitment at least as this concerns the demands the institutions place on families. And the key public institutions it invokes (e.g. public education and healthcare) are simply more generous and extensive versions of institutions that already exist in many contemporary liberal democracies. At any rate, I think the vision of a non-hierarchical society is both sufficiently realistic and sufficiently allied to the egalitarian commitments of Brighouse and Swift to challenge their skepticism about the harmony of family values and equality of opportunity. In a non-hierarchical society equality and family values can be realistically harmonized.

My third claim is more speculative. A valuable feature of Brighouse and Swift's book is that it is not an exercise in pure ideal theory. Their analysis is informed by contemporary sociological information about families and the challenges they face. It seeks to illuminate the nature and significance of family values in a way that might inform policy debates. This sensitivity to current political realities is in many ways a virtue but I suspect it subtly colors their interpretation of the relation between equality and family values. Contemporary societies are deeply hierarchical in ways that Brighouse, Swift and I find deeply objectionable. In the context of hierarchy most parents are, and have reason to be, anxious about their children's prospects. Many fear that unless they help their children 'get ahead', their children will be ill equipped to succeed in a highly competitive world in which their life prospects are uncertain and fragile. So those with the means send their children to elite schools and universities, they share their precious social capital with their children in a myriad of ways and they alert their children of the importance of out competing their rivals for scarce resources: college admissions, jobs, and homes. In our world, parental partiality frequently takes on an emulous dimension.

Moreover, emulous partiality is incentivized in hierarchical societies and it preys upon the natural concern that parents have for the well-being of their children. Brighouse and Swift are alive to this dynamic: 'When benefits are scarce, as they usually are, not everyone can get them. Parents who want their children to be among those who do get them will find themselves involved in the pursuit of competitive advantage; advantage over others is here valued instrumentally, as a means to the ultimate end of absolute benefit' (p. 134). Of course, as I have noted above, Brighouse and Swift are careful to deny that parents have a *right* to confer unfair advantages on their children. Their view is that legitimate pursuit of relationship goods by parents will have an inevitable but unintended consequence of disrupting equality of opportunity. And on their view: 'simply put, familial relationship goods are more important than fair equality of opportunity' (p. 143). My point is that the conclusion that family values and equality of opportunity collide is more reflective of the way in which family dynamics of hierarchal societies influence our political imagination than any deep tension between equality and relationship goods. We see how benignly motivated parental partiality under conditions of inequality can exacerbate injustice and we expect that dynamic to obtain, albeit in a less pronounced fashion, under conditions of equality. If I am right about the characteristics of a non-hierarchical society then this kind of inference, though tempting, is mistaken and should be resisted.

Conclusion

I have argued that fair equality of opportunity and relationship goods do not need to be balanced because, under hospitable conditions, they do not come into conflict. This is good news for egalitarianism because it shows that concern for the family cannot be enlisted in arguments against egalitarian justice. Yet as Brighouse and Swift suggest at various points, justice almost certainly requires more than fair equality of opportunity. Egalitarians have reason to be concerned not only with ensuring that the terms of competition for jobs and social positions are fair, but also with ensuring that people have fair access to familial goods and that the life prospects of all, irrespective of native endowment, are good. *Family Values* does not provide a full elaboration of a comprehensive egalitarian conception of justice but it illuminates the importance of familial relationship goods to such a conception.

Notes

1. References to page numbers for cited passages from the book appear in brackets.
2. To be sure, Brighouse and Swift (2014) think their analysis of the conflict between family relationship goods and fair equality of opportunity is relevant to guiding policy judgments in the actual, non-ideal world where the need to make tradeoffs between different values may arise in more dramatic ways. But their analysis purports also to reveal the tension between equality and family values that would obtain even in an ideally just world.
3. They also think that full implementation of fair equality of opportunity is likely to conflict with other values, including other dimensions of fairness. My concern here, however, is only with the purported conflict between fair equality of opportunity and family relationship goods.
4. See also Rawls (1971, p. 511) and Munoz-Darde (1999).
5. See Matthew Liao (2015) for a detailed treatment of the importance of love for children and its relevance to justice.
6. As I explain below, suitable political arrangements would include institutions that provide children with equal access to excellent education and healthcare as well as safe, secure housing in pleasant, well-provisioned neighborhoods with plenty of opportunities for recreation and leisure.
7. This does not mean that the state can never breach the privacy protections that are typically extended to families. Officials may reasonably be alert to signs of violence, abuse or neglect of children (or adults) in families and may, with suitable evidence and caution, intervene to address serious problems.
8. Brighouse and Swift do not offer an explicit articulation of what full realization of fair equality of opportunity would entail in terms of its effects on class hierarchies. But they do seem to assume that substantial inequalities between children and families would inevitably and legitimate arise even if the most egregious forms of unjust inequality that currently exist were eliminated. 'Suppose we eliminated economic inequalities between parents, or somehow insulated children's developmental opportunities from their influence. Different parents would still be members of different social networks; their friends and colleagues would be different – and unequally valuable as contacts, or sources of information, that could be used to help their children in the competition for the jobs and the qualifications helpful to achievement. Get rid of that cause of inequality in opportunities and parents will be unequally informed about the choices available to their children and which are the best means to their success. And information of that kind will be just a small part of the cultural capital that parents will remain able to convert into competitive advantage for their children – whether intentionally or inadvertently – as the unintended by-product of apparently innocuous interaction like bedtime stories and talk at family meals' (p. 29). Brighouse and Swift also anticipate that an economy that allows people to 'take responsibility for their own choices' (p. 30) would legitimately generate significant inequalities. The existence of such inequalities would presumably incentivize parents to try to secure competitive advantages for their own children.
9. Differences in the natural talents of children could be a source of inequality even if inequalities in developmental opportunities between children were eliminated or

effectively mitigated. As it is usually understood, fair equality of opportunity does not directly condemn inequalities that arise out of arbitrary differences in people's natural talents. I have not broached the issue of how such differences should be addressed in an egalitarian theory of justice. My own view is that differences in natural talents cannot justify significant inequalities in the overall life prospects of people. Of course, that view requires greater defense and elaboration than I can provide here. However, for the purposes of the analysis of this paper it is important to note that inequalities rooted in natural talents do not pose a special problem for the question of whether fair equality of opportunity inevitably collides with family values. The parenting strategies that different parents deploy in raising children do not affect the presence or absence of natural talents in children. So the family, as a social institution, is not itself a source in inequality grounded in natural talent. Of course, the resources and opportunities available to parents in raising children may significantly influence the degree to which children's talents are identified and cultivated.

Acknowledgements

I would like to thank Andrée-Anne Cormier, Anca Gheaus, Serena Olsaretti, Christine Sypnowich and an anonymous referee for helpful feedback on this paper.

Disclosure statement

No potential conflict of interest was reported by the author.

References

Brighouse, H., & Swift, A. (2014). *Family values: The ethics of parent-child relationships*. Princeton: Princeton University Press.
Liao, M. S. (2015). *The right to be loved*. Oxford: Oxford University Press.
Munoz-Darde, V. (1999). Is the family to be abolished then? *Proceedings of the Aristotelian Society, 99*(1), 37–56.
Rawls, J. (1971). *A theory of justice*. Cambridge, MA: Harvard University Press.
Rawls, J. (2001). *Justice as fairness: A restatement*. Cambridge, MA: Harvard University Press.

Flourishing children, flourishing adults: families, equality and the neutralism-perfectionism debate

Christine Sypnowich

ABSTRACT

Political philosophers are divided on the question of whether society should guide individuals in their projects and goals in light of the competing, yet overlapping, values of moral independence and human well-being. The lively neutralism-perfectionism debate appears to be significantly muted, however, when it comes to children who, all parties assume, should be guided by adults in their plans of life. Thus, in their stimulating new book, *Family Values: the Ethics of Parent-Child Relationships,* liberals Harry Brighouse and Adam Swift affirm the role of the family in directing and enabling children's flourishing. My paper challenges this distinction between parents and children in the liberal position to argue that the idea that it is appropriate to direct children to enable them to flourish, entails in fact, a commitment to policies that promote and enable the flourishing of all.

Introduction

The question of the extent to which society might guide individuals in their projects and goals is a point of contention among political philosophers, who are concerned about the weight to be given to the competing, yet overlapping, values of moral independence and human well-being. Perfectionists contend that the political community should seek to foster the living of excellent lives among its citizens. Most egalitarian political philosophers, however, are neutralist liberals, who contend that individuals should be left alone to choose how to live. They argue that the community treats its members as unequal (Dworkin, 1978, p. 132; Lecce, 2003, p. 538, 2008), or with disrespect (Quong, 2011, p. 7), or violates their autonomy (Rawls, 1971, p. 421; see also Rawls, 1993, pp. 173-211), if it uses public policy to improve human well-being. For neutralist liberals, the metric of distributive justice should be couched in terms of the means to individuals' ends, things that, as Rawls puts it, 'a rational man wants no matter what else he wants.' Questions of well-being should be relegated to the personal domain, congruent with state neutrality about the good. Under conditions of fair equality of opportunity, once goods are allocated according to a just principle of distribution, whether people flourish or not is taken to be a matter of their own responsibility; as Rawls puts it (1971, p. 94), 'it is assumed that the members of society are rational persons able to adjust their conceptions of the good to their situation.' Dworkin contends that neutrality follows from the ideal of equality: showing equal concern and respect to people requires that one be neutral about individuals' plans of life. The 'beer-drinking, television-watching' citizen's ideas about how to live should not count for less than that of the intellectual or the aesthete. 'A liberal theory of equality rules out ... appeal to the inherent value of one theory of what is good in life' and the economic market is a particularly apt model where the state plays no role in determining people's options (1978, p. 132).[1]

An exception to the neutralist view is typically made for children. Mill famously articulated the idea that 'the only purpose for which power can be rightfully exercised over any member of a civilised community, against his will, is to prevent harm to others,' but with the caveat that his doctrine 'is meant to apply only to human beings in the maturity of their faculties' (1966, p. 14). Rawls notes (1971, p. 249) that his model of justice does not apply to children or those who 'cannot rationally advance their interest.' The resolute neutralist Barry, who argues (1995, p. 216) that 'principles of justice' should not be deployed 'to address other moral questions,' contends that citizens undertake the education of children to provide them with the 'opportunity to live better lives' or to 'live well' (Barry, 2001, pp. 221–224).

The idea of liberty for adults, paternalism for children, is almost standard in liberal political philosophy. Most liberals note that given differences in capacities for rational choice track maturity, generational inequality in the matter of perfectionist paternalism is no injustice, but an exception that proves the rule. Indeed inherent in the charge of 'paternalism' made by liberals against perfectionism is that the state is inappropriately acting like a parent acts towards a child; whilst paternalism is appropriate for the asymmetrical relationships of families and schools, it is wrong for the relationship between the coercive state and its adult citizens. Quong thus couches his neutralist position in these terms: a perfectionist politics means the state treats citizens 'as if they lack the ability to make effective choices about their own lives' (2011, p. 106).[2]

This paper challenges the distinction in the liberal neutralist position, wherein perfectionist policies for children are permitted, but perfectionist policies for adults are not. Many will anticipate the familiar critique of this distinction, which takes a 'children's liberation' stance, making the case that children should be treated as self-governing and emancipated from paternalist strictures.[3] On this view, children should join adults within the neutralist framework that leaves individuals alone to make their own choices. This approach has had influence in debates about political indoctrination in schools. Liberals have considered how to impart a civic education to children in which they are inculcated in the values of citizenship without being given a particular liberal (or conservative) political script.[4] Some liberals propose severe strictures on the extent to which even parents can impart their conceptions of value to their children, given the importance of autonomous choice (Callan, 2002, 127–130).[5]

My argument, however, takes the opposite tack. Whilst I am prepared to agree with the children's liberationists that young people's capacity for autonomy is too often underestimated, I contend that the community should seek to provide guidance in the choices made by everyone, children and adults, to enable people to flourish. I argue that this is the right conclusion to draw from recent exciting work being done by political philosophers on the ethics of the family, such as the stimulating new book, *Family Values: The Ethics of Parent-Child Relationships*, by Harry Brighouse and Adam Swift, in which they invoke the criterion of children's flourishing to defend parents' childrearing practices. I contend that the idea that it is appropriate to direct children to enable them to flourish entails, in fact, a commitment to policies that enable the flourishing of all. I conclude therefore that reflection on the value of the family and the well-being of its members demonstrates the power of an 'egalitarian flourishing' approach to social justice that departs from the neutralist orthodoxy in political philosophy.

The flourishing family

The starting point of *Family Values* is how the institution of the family is in tension with a commitment to social equality. The book notes that unjust advantages and disadvantages are conferred on children who grow up in different family structures, and contends that there should be limitations on parental partiality (e.g. all things being equal, not providing one's children with elite private schooling) so children are not unduly burdened or benefitted by the parents they happen to have. There is now a large literature on the question of how the 'affective family,' as Macleod (2002, p. 213) puts it, can be reconciled with egalitarian principles. It is incontrovertible that there are contingent – and unjust – disparities in competence, commitment and resources from one set of parents to the next. Yet the benefits accrued through family relationships (manifest in Brighouse and Swift's much-cited example, reading bedtime stories, which are also a key factor in improving children's life prospects), and moreover, the non-fungibility of the benefits of the family via other institutional arrangements, means that the rearing of children by their parents is nonetheless the ideal.

This is a persuasive argument, which makes obvious that the well-being of parents, too, is tied up with participating in, and enabling, the well-being of their children. As Brighouse and Swift incisively put it, for 'a child's interests to be reliably met,' she needs to be 'cared for by at least one adult who loves her,' an adult who finds 'herself experiencing the parent-child relationship as a source of joy and satisfaction in the way most helpful to the child's development' (2014, pp. 72–73). They thus concur with Brennan (2014) and Gheaus (2015) that parents have a duty to provide 'intrinsic' or 'special' goods of childhood, coining the phrase 'relationship goods' as what is special about family life. As they state it baldly (2014, p. 74), 'it is valuable *for children* that the adults who raise them enjoy the relationship.' Adults benefit from the child-parent relationship and it is right that they should do so, for the sake of children's fundamental interests.

This approach is in keeping with Brighouse's educational views (2006, ch. 3), where he acknowledges the influence of perfectionist argument in his claim that education should be 'for flourishing,' to 'prepare children to live flourishing lives.' Schools' curriculum should take a stand on what counts as a valuable life and develop children's capacity for well-being, by enabling them to form meaningful personal relationships, to find value in nature and works of beauty, to become physically fit and enjoy physical activity and recreation, and to nurture their intellectual and critical faculties. But although Brighouse deploys the flourishing idea in the case of children, elsewhere (2004, p. 72) he is assiduously austere in his conception of the state's role in promoting conceptions of the good among adults, arguing that the state should avoid being 'excessively perfectionistic' by operating under a 'neutrality constraint' wherein the state is neutral regarding citizens' plans of life, a constraint that has severe implications, calling into question, for example, state subsidies for the arts (Brighouse, 1995, p. 41).

In his introductory book on political philosophy, Swift elaborates (2006, p. 159) the difference between perfectionism and neutralism, hypothesising that a perfectionist would be prepared to promote 'family values' on the grounds, for example, that stable heterosexual marriages are intrinsically better for people, a reason that would be ruled out by neutralists (and, I would add, in fact most perfectionists!). Swift goes on to speculate, provocatively, that it may be possible, however, for the neutral state to promote the traditional family if it could be argued that 'other family forms are more likely to harm the children raised in them.'

In *Family Values,* the authors seem at first to have no truck with perfectionism for adult citizens in the liberal community: adults' flourishing is important only insofar as it is instrumental to the flourishing of children. But Brighouse and Swift make an additional move, and defend the institution of the family as a site for human well-being for both generations. They draw on Nussbaum's conception of the many constituents of human functioning, from bodily health to play and leisure, to say that children have a right to parents who are best placed to provide them with these goods (2014, p. 60), and moreover that adults have a right to become parents in order to avail themselves of those goods unique to family relationships that contribute to their own flourishing. In cultivating children's capacities, parents find a unique source of human well-being, and this consideration has independent weight. Barring neglect or abuse, adults have a right to parent or what Clayton calls (2006, p. 57) 'the right to rear' the children they procreate (Brighouse & Swift, 2014, p. 110). Thus, Brighouse and Swift find themselves invoking perfectionist arguments in their case for the value of family relationships for both children and parents. The result is an original, compelling and incisive analysis of the family, replete with common sense, which judiciously affirms the special contribution of childrearing in families to human well-being, whilst acknowledging and seeking to mitigate the injustices this inevitably entails.

However, there are some puzzling aspects to this account. The authors' idea of relationship goods invites a comparison with primary goods, Rawls's all-purpose goods of instrumental value for unspecified projects and goals. For Rawls, the state should not set out what is intrinsically valuable, a position that we saw Brighouse, and possibly the avowedly liberal Swift (Mulhall & Swift, 1997, p. xxii), seem to endorse elsewhere. The only possible exception is a liberal one: autonomy is a 'central value' for human life (Mulhall and Swift, p. 250), which is potentially at risk in the intimate relations of parents with their children (Brighouse & Swift, 2003, p. 369).

What, then, is the status of the intrinsically valuable relationship goods in this liberal picture? And if the state is obligated to safeguard these goods by refraining from socialising childrearing, why stop there? Why not protect, promote and nurture other valuable goods for human beings? These questions arise given the egalitarian framework of the book's argument. It seems an uneasy conclusion that the commitment to distributive justice must be qualified to allow families to transmit goods which are readily acknowledged as sources of unjust 'social reproduction' that reinforce disparities of social class and position. Brighouse and Swift thus emphasise the importance of 'anti-poverty measures' to mitigate the injustice of inter-family inequality. If people have a right to parent, 'a positive right to familial relationship goods,' this means the state should attend to 'a social environment that allows the parent's relationship with her child to be more than the struggle for life's necessities' (Brighouse & Swift, 2014, p. 148). They go so far as to say that these goods should be conceived as 'distribuenda' whose distribution is 'massively' affected by public policy.

The latter point is particularly congenial if, as I argue, we should consider distributive justice more generally as a matter of aiming for the equality of flourishing, where what is being distributed is not goods, income or resources, but the constituents of living well (see Sypnowich, 2014, 2017). Social policies like mandating flexible arrangements at work for parents, home visits to help with all facets of childrearing, even, perhaps, workshops on reading bedtime stories presuppose an 'egalitarian flourishing' view, whereby the political community that seeks greater equality is committed to enabling people to live well. Neutralists might object that whilst parents may inculcate particular conceptions of the good in their children, the state may not do so. However, the task of enabling children to flourish inevitably involves the political community in, not just the provision of public education, but also in the support needed for families to enjoy relationship goods.

On my egalitarian flourishing view, it is possible to promote the relationship goods of the family and also attend to social inequality by means of a single approach that focuses on human well-being. Unequal distribution of wealth can have the effect that some people are poorly housed, badly nourished, ill educated, or uncultured, among other things. Inequality is a social ill because of the damage it does to the lives people live. Resources or property are relevant therefore insofar as they contribute to how people fare under one distribution or another.[6] Ultimately, the answer to the question, 'equality of what?' is flourishing, since whatever policies or principles we adopt, it is flourishing, or well-being, a metric that cannot be elucidated without reference to the objectively valuable, which we hope will be made more equal as a result of our endeavours.

Family Values seems to make moves towards such an approach. However, in their conclusion, Brighouse and Swift wring their hands about the potentially alarming perfectionist implications of their view. They concede that government could not be 'entirely neutral' if it took their arguments to heart, but they reassure their gentle readers (2014, p. 178) that they of course do not intend 'a single, monistic, vision of how people should live their lives as a whole.' Devoted and happy dads though they are, not everyone need subscribe to their ideal of the good life. Moreover, they back away from some of their earlier arguments – suggesting, for example, that readers could take from their book only advice about the proper limits to parental partiality in childrearing, and leave behind the larger political claims. They also propose (2014, p. 180) that the case for protecting relationship goods for the sake of adults' flourishing can be jettisoned from their account, or conceived as simply compensating for the bias against successful parenting given the costs of juggling work and family life are 'unduly high' in today's societies. This is a theme that they broached in an earlier essay (2006, p. 108), where they suggested that 'existing arrangements' might be 'biased against parenting in a way that would justify pro-family policies as consistent with an egalitarian or neutralist conception of distributive justice.'

Thus human flourishing emerges as a somewhat provisional and fraught value in the argument. On the one hand, the family is affirmed as an institution that enables the flourishing of children, which in turn depends on the flourishing of adults, and further still, the flourishing of adults is something that is inherently important and worth protecting. On the other hand, the only goods on deck are the relationship goods of the family, and moreover, adults' enjoyment of relationship goods that is constitutive of their flourishing turns out to be a throwaway argument. The paternalism bugbear is such that there is no role for a general view about the context for human flourishing where the political community should provide the conditions or opportunities that would facilitate flourishing in all its dimensions.

However, if the flourishing of children is our aim, we will need to liberate ourselves from the characteristically American wariness of state regulation with which Brighouse and Swift, surprisingly, seem burdened. For all their appreciation of the role of family relationships as a source of human flourishing for both children and adults, and the role of the state in safeguarding these relationships, Brighouse and Swift are at pains to contrast their position with perfectionist views that they caricature as being 'made to act on the judgements of others,' or to be 'coerced or manipulated' (2014, pp. 178, 61).

It is not possible, in fact, to work with a premiss about human flourishing for children and then deny its operation for individuals upon adulthood. We cannot dispatch ideas of fostering adult well-being in our society with the view, as Brighouse puts it (2006, p. 43), that 'we should not, as a general matter, presume that we know better than other people how they should best lead their lives.' The argument about the rearing and education of children falls down unless it presupposes a fact of the matter – however pluralistic and non-coercive – about living well and the proper role of the state in promoting it. This suggests that equality is not simply a matter of individuals' access to material goods but also, the well-being individuals derive from such goods, and moreover, the well-being that comes from other goods.

Dimensions of living well

There are several reasons why the argument for the flourishing of children presupposes a general and substantive commitment to the flourishing of adults. First, I have stressed in this paper that what is bad about being poor is not simply having less money than other people, but also deprivation of the constituents of a valuable life. Thus, in attending to child poverty, the community seeks to provide, not just additional family income, but opportunities for flourishing, in the form of children-oriented supplements to the welfare state such as school dinners, free tickets to the theatre, or opportunities for sport or recreation. And the idea of a valuable life for children cannot be severed from such an idea for adults, where nutrition, culture and fitness figure as aspects of a live well lived.

Second, the project of preparing for flourishing cannot be hived off from adult flourishing insofar as we need to identify what adult flourishing looks like in order to equip children for it. Indeed, Brighouse and Swift themselves (2014, p. 84) put their project in terms of stipulating that 'in order to develop into flourishing adults,' children should be raised in loving families. If we take a perfectionist position about genuine sources of value that children are to be inculcated to develop and achieve, then we need to identify what those sources of value are. We say that children need to be loved, they need to develop their talents, and that they need to become autonomous. All this is to prepare them for lives that we suppose ought to take a certain form, whereby adults with fulfilling lives are in loving relationships, engaged in activities that make the most of their abilities, and are self-directed in their plans and projects. Thus, we are working with a conception of a flourishing adult life for which children are being prepared.

Third, we need to ensure that we provide the ongoing conditions that make it possible for these young flourishing beings to be able to actualise the capacities that parents' practices and our systems of education have nourished and fostered. Many educational theorists are rightly wary of 'education for training,' arguing that education is better conceived in a more holistic sense of developing our personhood, exemplified in Oakeshott's idea of inculcation into the 'conversation of mankind' (Bakhurst, 2016, 2011, p. 159). Nonetheless education is of course preparation for something that awaits the child; that is, a community that provides rich opportunities for flourishing. It would be odd to cultivate capacities for intellectual inquiry, loving relationships and the appreciation of nature in young people, and then shrug our shoulders at the fact that the options that await them upon adulthood are skewed towards the values of reality shows and Facebook, the porn-fed relationships of hooking up and sexting, the leisure pursuits of online shopping and hanging out at the mall.

Indeed, there is an implicit commitment to ensuring that the community is so constituted that adults have chosen paths that are of genuine value that children may follow. For all the neutralism of mainstream political theory, most liberal societies seek to promote valuable ways of living, manifest in such policies as funding for the arts, subsidised adult education, heritage conservation, the preservation of green spaces, from national wilderness areas to city parks (interestingly, much perfectionist public policy is to be found at the local level). Moreover, we also hope that in educating children to prepare them for flourishing, they will grow up to foster those constituents of a flourishing life more generally in their society, be it contributing to culture, undertaking life-long learning or participating in the civic life of their communities.

Fourth, education and childrearing is therefore not just a matter of providing skills. A common view is that students are being given tools, or capacities, that are merely instrumental to their plans of life, rather than being directed to particular plans. Education is thus a kind of proactive effort at giving children 'all purpose means,' analogous to Rawls's idea of primary goods as what rational individuals want 'no matter what else' they want. Thus neutralists might object to my argument with the view that paternalism for children is quite proper, but it is justified by a neutral approach based on fair equality of opportunity which permits intervention in their lives only to resource them, e.g. with minimum levels of nutrition, or mandatory schooling, for whatever projects they decide to undertake. Even being 'raised in loving families' is thus a neutral instrumental good to be protected by the neutral state.

Preparing for flourishing, however, means equipping children with capacities that are not merely a means to some undetermined end; they are, rather, constitutive of what it is to live well. In his philosophy of education (2011, p. 159),

Bakhurst stresses that the task of acculturating children is to enable 'autonomy and the opportunity to live a worthwhile life,' to allow them 'to engage in productive work, to benefit from satisfying leisure and to enjoy happy relationships with others.' Brighouse (2006, pp. 43–45) also counsels that parents and teachers should be guided by judgements about a student's general and particular interests that will 'tend to her long-term flourishing' with a substantive view of the constituents of that flourishing. *Family Values* (2014, pp. 70, 60) affirms that childrearing aims at children's 'weighty interests' in, not just 'future agency' but also well-being per se, adducing, as noted above, a detailed list of the constituents of that well-being. Taking a substantive view on well-being requires, of course, a pluralistic approach; there are many diverse ways to live well, and parents and schools must tailor both childrearing and education to suit individual children's abilities and dispositions.

Thus when children study Shakespeare, for example, they are of course acquiring a host of 'transferable skills,' to use today's education jargon. They improve their reading comprehension and vocabulary, and they acquire knowledge of literature, history, and a grasp of human culture that will help them in whatever paths they choose in life. But it would do violence to the learning of Shakespeare to reduce it to a simply instrumental exercise. Becoming familiar with the works of Shakespeare is intrinsically valuable; it enriches children's lives and contributes to their flourishing, and will, parents and educators hope, play a similar role in their adult lives too.

Brighouse and Swift contend that 'one might plausibly deny that government policy may properly promote adults' interest in parenting' (2014, 179) and thus some pro-family policies can be justified solely in terms of their benefits for children, even if they indirectly benefit their adult caregivers. However, if we are cowed by such neutralist squeamishness we end up with a very odd picture of social policy, where, for example, their recommendations of 'policies to combat poverty, to socialise the costs of children's education and health care, and to help…parents achieve better work-life balance' resolutely avoid any reference to how people's lives go better if they are assisted in the rearing of their children.

An example of existing perfectionist policy for adults are the social benefits that accrue to people if they marry or have children, in terms of tax relief or state subsidies. Indeed, welfare state policies such as the family allowance were the response to, not just instrumental calculations of ensuring the existence of future workforces, or even the important goal of reducing child poverty. They also emerged from a view about how stable relationships with life partners and children were constituents of human well-being. The architects of Western welfare states were specifically concerned with how family life was good for their citizens, both children and adults (Beveridge, 1943, pp. 16, 54, 125; Blake, 2009, pp. 91–94, 112; see also Macedo, 2015, pp. 80–83).

Living well

The constituents of a valuable life can be grouped into three categories. There is the ability to choose how to live since, as all liberals should agree, a non-autonomous life falls short as a flourishing existence. Another constituent of well-being is objectively worthwhile pursuits, for there are better and worse ways of living and even the freely chosen pursuit can be defective. Finally, personal contentment is an important feature of flourishing, since freely chosen objective pursuits are inadequate sources of well-being if the person derives no pleasure or fulfilment from them. As Sher puts it (1997, p. 229), 'we can hardly deny that happiness, pleasure, and enjoyment are among life's goods.' Though the valuable does not necessarily produce pleasure, this should not entail an austere version of perfectionism where pleasure figures as 'an accretion' relevant only insofar as worthy pursuits tend to produce it (Hurka, 1996, p. 26).

How much weight to give each component is a tricky question; these things are impossible to measure precisely and there will be trade-offs, though one would cease to count as flourishing if any one component is too lacking. Contentment, for example, might be thought worth sacrificing for a life of struggle – the tortured genius example comes to mind. But no general position can be made for giving any one constituent priority over the others. This is to be settled particularistically, given different persons' circumstances, aptitudes, plans and personalities.

This conception of has classical philosophical antecedents. For Aristotle, happiness or eudaimonia refers to the idea of fulfilling our capacities: activity, using our reason, in the pursuit of excellence. The ancient Greek conception of 'the good life' is clearly a long way from the hedonist conception promoted by beer commercials and popular culture, but Aristotle (2000, pp. 139–140) certainly believed contentment was a feature of eudaimonia, the Greek understanding of happiness as consisting in living well, if not its aim: 'the happy person therefore also needs bodily goods, external goods and good fortune.' Marx's conception of species being (1978, pp. 87–88), wherein individuals self-actualise through labour, understood as free, creative activity, is similar in its emphasis on active engagement and the development of human potential, but also his view that properly ordered, labour produces a feeling of well-being.[7]

It follows that well-being involves more than the satisfaction of biological needs. Here, I concur with Brighouse and Swift that Nussbaum's list (2000, p. 75) is instructive, though for both adults and children, who need food, shelter, and health, but also education, friendship and love, participation in public life, play and sport, experiences of nature, culture and opportunities for intellectual reflection in order to enjoy well-being. Improvements in well-being derived from cultural, aesthetic and social pursuits are indeed likely more important than improvements in physical well-being, once a threshold of some kind has been met (Griffin, 1986, pp. 52–53).[8] A society which treats its members justly, and thus seeks to render them materially equal, should therefore focus on human flourishing and look to, not just the family, but a variety of social forms, institutions and a plethora of constituents of human well-being, as vehicles for egalitarian policy.

Autonomy, choice and flourishing

Brighouse and Swift's unease with a potentially illiberal perfectionist approach centres on a concern for respect for human agency, to 'be the author of one's own life,' where we accept people's judgements about their own good as authoritative (2014, p. 61). The idea that public institutions should enable the flourishing of citizens and that egalitarianism should be understood as seeking to equalise flourishing, runs up against the objection that this involves violating people's autonomy. On this view, adults should be free to choose how to live without the state coercing, or even seeking to influence, their choices. Here, I offer a few thoughts to counter this idea.

Perfectionist policy tends to be put in simplistic terms, as though our ways of life must be either immune to influence or putty in the hands of others. My view eschews coercion as incompatible with the autonomy that is essential to human flourishing, and appreciates the diverse sources of living well; it is thus pluralist, not unitary, about the good. Thus, in contrast to the narrow focus of some liberal accounts, autonomy does not figure as the singular good to be promoted to the exclusion of all others. The expression 'the good' pastiched in much neutralist literature is highly misleading; there are many, diverse and incommensurable ways of living well. Football is as much a contender as opera for human well-being, and there is a case for equalising access to both. This is particularly evident in how most parents understand the flourishing of their children, seeking to introduce them to a variety of valuable pursuits and pastimes so that they may find their own particular good.

Anti-perfectionists complain that perfectionist subsidies or taxes 'artificially distort the opportunity costs in people's choices,' (Lecce, 2008, pp. 122–123, 134) and fail to treat individuals with respect (Quong, 2011, p. 16).[9] But such views involve a false understanding of the nature of agency, wherein individuals are only freely choosing if untouched by social influences. One certainly lives a better life if one is 'leading it from the inside, according to my beliefs about value' (Kymlicka, 2002, p. 216), and people's lives cannot be made better 'against their own convictions' (Dworkin, 2000, p. 268). A conviction is not a conviction unless it is one's own, and one cannot live any other way but from the 'inside.' But the person 'on the inside,' her needs, desires and tastes, are shaped by her situation on the outside, the many influences of a social milieu.

A modest 'social thesis' that understands that persons are inevitably influenced by their environment is thus an important corrective to misconceptions about choice. The idea of responsiveness to reasons, at the heart of our ideal of autonomy, means that persons, young and old, are not pure will, but are beings responsive to external sources of information and judgement. Our friends, parents, or those with authority, as well as education and important life experiences, all contribute to our ideas about how to live.[10] And this does not cease when one grows up or leaves school.

Many of the factors that influence our choices also come from advertising, product differentiation, brand promotions or marketing, and are not conducive to choices made on the basis of reasons. Indeed, the market, often assumed to support the neutralism of the liberal state because its exchanges are conducted without state direction, in fact makes for quite significant consequences for the kinds of values one pursues. And human flourishing is often adversely affected, even measured on a simple scale of expressions of satisfaction. Furthermore, markets can shape our choices without being held to public account or democratic control. That neutralist positions continue to evoke the 'marketplace of ideas' seems both misleading and naïve.

Kymlicka, for example, argues for 'social perfectionism' over 'state perfectionism' and deploys the metaphor of a 'cultural marketplace' to defend the 'free association of individuals' who share cultures or good ways of life, unfettered by state interference (2002, pp. 246–248). This position is at odds with Kymlicka's multiculturalist views; in his argument for special rights for minority cultures, he in fact rejects the possibility of the neutral 'cultural marketplace,' taking the position that the state must correct for those conditions that disadvantage some in the pursuit of valuable ways of life (1995, p. 113).[11] Furthermore, in his recent work on animals with Donaldson (2013, p. 34), Kymlicka explicitly invokes the goal of enabling the flourishing of non-human species.

However, when it comes to human goods that are vulnerable or threatened such as access to natural wilderness areas or historical artefacts, Kymlicka argues (2002, p. 247) that the state should offer support, not because these are valuable options that contribute to human flourishing, but for the sake of neutrality, seeking to offset 'wear and tear' so that they are available for future individuals. 'Even if the cultural marketplace can be relied on to ensure that existing people can identify valuable ways of life, it cannot be relied on to ensure that future people have a valuable range of options.' Dworkin's approach is similar; he suggests (1985, p. 232) that funding for the arts is permitted given the role of culture in providing 'complex and diverse' cultural forms, thus society should, as 'trustees for the future complexity of our own culture,' protect the 'structure of our intellectual culture' rather than 'particular aesthetic events.'[12]

However, this contrast between, on the one hand, identifying the good, the province of the cultural marketplace, and on the other, preserving the options markets produce, is unhelpful. The reasons to think that the market will fail to preserve the valuable are also the reasons to think the market will fail to make the valuable available in the first place. The market's problems are not just limited to inequalities of distribution, as Dworkin assumes in his market-based egalitarianism. Thus, the political community can only ensure a 'valuable range of options' if it also determines what the valuable, however plural, might be. After all, there will be many vulnerable options, and not all of them can or should be protected. Perfectionism is part and parcel of the 'conserving options strategy' – both for funding for the arts, and for protecting family values against forces, from poverty to high-flying careers, that can undermine parents' relationships with their children. Talk of conserving options presupposes a perfectionist premiss about the thing that is to be protected: in this case, the 'distinctively valuable' character of the family in the face of adverse forces against it (Brighouse & Swift, 2006, p. 107).

It seems inevitable that protecting the valuable entails action that counteracts the market and what one economist (Offer, 2006, p. 74) calls its 'myopic bias.' Given the pernicious forces at work affecting choice, encouraging worthwhile choices – be they the relationship goods of the family, valuable cultural pursuits, or the connections that are forged within neighbourhoods and local communities – is a legitimate balancing measure.[13] Why not, as Sher puts it (1997, p. 73), 'take (benign) advantage of a causal process that would occur anyhow?'

Moreover, in an age of sophisticated communications, the astonishing mobility of capital and consumption has sometimes meant a greater variety of cultural forms, but more often it has produced an increasing homogeneity, as more and more of the world's population consumes the same fast food, hums the same popular songs, and wears the same casual clothing. If sameness is considered equality, this might be thought of as the measure of some political ideal, but our argument has stressed the importance of pluralism in any adequate conception of equality. Counteracting the market is also important in light of an appreciation for self-determination, whereby meaningful choice, not just consumer's choice in a context of market options, is intrinsic to an autonomous life. I thus find congenial recent proposals (Sunstein, 2014, pp. 137–138) that 'helpful choice architecture' should structure the inevitable context of choice to 'nudge' us to make good choices and enhance our choice-making capacity, given human beings' limitations of time, interest and attention.

Public provision of opportunities for family life and social interaction can be seen therefore as an equalising policy; indeed, such opportunities are much more important than affluence in making a person content. This is reported by scholars in the discipline of 'Happiness Studies' bordering psychology and economics, who stress the surprising connection between feelings of satisfaction and the choice of valuable pursuits such as walking rather than driving, or seeing friends and spending time with family rather than shopping or watching television (Frank, 1999; Gilbert, 2007; Layard, 2005; Nettle, 2006; Offer, 2006; Victor, 2008). We should be wary of 'being seduced by over-simplified conceptions of happiness as a matter of "feeling good"', since living life in 'all its fullness' often involves struggle or exertion, not pleasure per se (Smith, 2009, p. 202), but much of the recent literature provides evidence to suggest that 'the good life' has less to do with the hedonism of the beer commercial and more to do with the Aristotlean conception of exertion and fulfilment than one might have thought.

The family is a perfect example of this. As Brighouse and Swift make clear, it involves conflict, anxiety and struggle, just as much as it rewards its members with love, support, and even joy. Relationship goods are thus examples of all three constituents of flourishing; they are the object of brute subjective preferences and the means for developing autonomy; they are sources of happiness and satisfaction; and they are objectively worthwhile. Expanding on the insights of *Family Values*, a flourishing approach to distributive justice should adopt policies to resource those families that are disadvantaged in their ability to foster relationship goods.

Of course, children's capacity to flourish can be adversely or positively influenced by factors beyond the community's control – e.g. to be raised by an ill-tempered parent, or a parent who confronts personal or medical challenges, or whose parents engage in a bitter divorce, or whose parents' life plans conflict with those of the child. Parents can be poor at their role and family relationships can be dysfunctional and unhappy. Given these diverse, contingent and to some extent irremediable factors, public policy cannot ensure that children's flourishing is strictly equal. But these considerations are not unique to children; indeed, the challenges confronted by children's parents indicate that adults, too, will face obstacles to flourishing that cannot be wholly eliminated by political action. Nonetheless, the seriousness of these potential problems in family life suggests that the case for the involvement of the political community is particularly important. Families and schools should have a bipartite relationship that seeks the well-being of children. Remedy for shortfalls in functioning is in part a community effort, and the community should seek to provide resources to help children – and their parents – whose family circumstances are not ideal. A flourishing approach does not pressure parents to produce 'perfect children,' arguably already a phenomenon of the culture of the contemporary family, where hyper-ambitious parents 'helicopter' their offspring and micro-manage children's lives to ensure worldly success. Rather, the community is responsible for providing support and assistance to take the pressure off parents who might find it hard to cope with the challenges of childrearing for all kinds of reasons.

It might be objected that even if schools prepare students for flourishing, this is the consequence of a myriad of private decisions made in families about the kind of schooling children should be given, and thus the political community's role in the flourishing enterprise is rightly rather limited. However, the model of public education reflects the principle that the political community should have significant authority over children's flourishing. What students are taught in schools is a matter of public concern, and thus curriculum is decided in light of government decisions about what is needed for students to have the requisite tools for citizenship, basic skills for work, but also more ambitiously, the constituents of flourishing, such as autonomy. Of course, parents have input into this, and where a community does not engage parents sufficiently, innovations in curriculum can precipitate crises of legitimacy (in Ontario, government took a 'go it alone' approach to liberalise sex education which has precipitated a predictable backlash from conservative parents). Even private schools, much as they seek to evade the strictures of public authority, must ensure their students meet state-stipulated educational requirements (although, as Swift has argued, private education is difficult to justify if one believes in equality). Thus, for all the input from parents and families, the state acts as an independent coercive agent to ensure the well-being of children and can thereby facilitate the community's egalitarian goals.

In sum, the redistributive mechanisms of the welfare state, conjoined with a number of local policies, are important devices for improving and equalising flourishing. The public school system has potential as an important vehicle for equality, not just in its curriculum, but as community hubs, the site of accessible activities to foster the flourishing of families, be it through workshops, nature walks, theatre and other events after school hours, or as a conduit for the distribution of aids that can support family life.[14] Moreover, a theme worth exploring further, schools themselves could model the relations of equality, and instil the values of egalitarian flourishing in their classrooms, to compensate for the inequality too often generated by family life. All this would serve to improve human flourishing, for children, to equip them for flourishing lives, and also to improve the flourishing of all family members, for whom many goods, including relationship goods, are crucial sources of human well-being.

Conclusion

In perhaps an ironic gesture, the appealing cover of Brighouse and Swift's excellent book is taken from a Norman Rockwell painting that depicts an American family gathered around the dinner table. Well-being exudes from the faces of all, young and old. There is no need for a caveat that the state should be agnostic about the good, or that the family is an option that has no special place in the menu of life choices. This reflects the practices of our liberal political communities that in fact recognise the value of the family, and seek to support it in a variety of social welfare institutions, tax structures, and the public policies of neighbourhood design. Brighouse and Swift's powerful argument for why families are valuable, given the intrinsically valuable relationship goods rightly enjoyed by all their members, makes it clear that political philosophy has been impoverished for its jettisoning of questions of human flourishing. It is high time political philosophers liberated themselves from the unfortunate neutralist baggage of Rawlsian liberalism and acknowledged how the promotion of flourishing undergirds much progressive social policy in a variety of domains. If we are to enable children to live flourishing lives, we will need to appreciate the importance of family values, as Brighouse and Swift so persuasively argue. And thereby we will need to elaborate, more generally, life values, the constituents of human flourishing in all dimensions, and an egalitarian political philosophy that centres on enabling flourishing for all.

Notes

1. Dworkin does admit that the market has inegalitarian aspects, too, insofar as some are disadvantaged in their ability to participate in the market.
2. Though Quong (2011, pp. 301–305) argues that children should be educated in the values of a liberal democracy.
3. Firestone (1970) is perhaps the most famous exponent of this view, who conceives the liberation of children as part and parcel of women's liberation; see also Adams et al. (1971).
4. Gutman (1987) provides the classic contemporary liberal argument for public provision of civic education as the 'conscious social reproduction' of democratic values. See also Galston (1989, pp. 89–102). Levinson (1999, pp. 36–50) extends the argument to include a 'weakly perfectionist' duty on the part of schools to inculcate autonomy in children as the responsibility of the liberal political community. But see also Waldren (2013).
5. Brighouse and Swift qualify this to some extent in their 'relationship goods' account (2014, ch. 6).
6. I am following Parfit (2000) in his insistence that egalitarianism must be premissed on a person-affecting claim.
7. Thus Marx (1978, pp. 87–88) speaks of how the transcendence of private property brings with it the 'emancipation of all human senses.' I explore the role of Marx's ideas for a conception of equality focussed on human flourishing in Sypnowich (2003).
8. G. A. Cohen's ideal of community (2008, ch. 1), where justice requires individuals being prepared to contribute for the sake of the satisfaction of needs other than their own, suggests individuals care not just about who has what, but how they are doing with their respective shares, whether they are able to derive fulfilment from their share of resources.
9. Conly (2012, p. 16) contends that autonomy has been 'overvalued' and that the state should interfere with autonomy in order to prevent harm.
10. The idea of the social constitution of the self has had wide influence in philosophy; for a sample of views see Bakhurst & Sypnowich, 1995.
11. Kymlicka's contention that the doctrine of neutral justification, precisely because of its non-neutral effects, ill-serves minority groups has prompted Patten (2014, p. 115) to come to the doctrine's rescue with a version based on 'neutrality of treatment,' whereby 'the state's policies must be equally accommodating of rival conceptions of the good.'
12. This position is subjected to criticism from fellow neutralists. As noted above, Brighouse (1995, p. 63) concludes that if liberals want to justify funding for the arts, they may have to give up 'the neutrality constraint.' Quong (2011, pp. 90–91) bites the bullet and insists that demand should dictate the provision of cultural goods, which should be paid for 'at the point of consumption' by those who avail themselves of such goods.
13. Arneson puts this provocatively (2003, 213): 'one does not exhibit disrespect for a person by treating her in accordance with principles that she actually rejects, but that she would accept if she were fully rational.'

14. Where I live the unsuccessful campaign to save our downtown high school centred on, not just children's education, but also the school's contribution to community life and human well-being more generally.

Acknowledgements

For very helpful comments on earlier versions of this essay, I would like to thank Omar Bachour, Harry Brighouse, Jeremy Butler, Jan Derry, Kyle Johannsen, Ryan McSheffrey, David Miller, Judith Suissa, Adam Swift, John White, Patricia White, and participants at the following: the Political Theory Workshop at Nuffield College, Oxford, the Institute of Education Philosophy Seminar at University College London, and the *Family Values* panel at the 2015 European Consortium for Political Research meetings. In particular, I am grateful to Andrée-Anne Cormier, David Bakhurst, Meira Levinson and Danielle Zwarthoed, for their detailed and generous feedback.

Disclosure statement

No potential conflict of interest was reported by the author.

References

Adams, P., Berg, L., Berger, N., Duane, M., Neill, A.S., & Ollendorf, R. (1971). *Children's rights: Toward the liberation of the child*. New York, NY: Praeger.

Aristotle. (2000). In R. Crisp (Ed.), *Nichomachean ethics*. Cambridge: Cambridge University Press.

Arneson, R. (2003). Liberal neutrality on the good: An autopsy. In S. Wall & G. Klosko (Eds.), *Perfectionism and neutrality: Essays in liberal theory* (pp. 191–218). Lanham, MD: Rowman and Littlefield.

Bakhurst, D. (2011). *The formation of reason*. London: Wiley-Blackwell.

Bakhurst, D. (2016). Education and conversation. In D. Bakhurst & P. Fairfield (Eds.), *Education and conversation: Exploring Oakeshott's legacy* (pp. 5–25). London: Bloomsbury.

Bakhurst, D., & Sypnowich, C. (Eds.). (1995). *The social self*. London: Sage.

Barry, B. (1995). *Justice as impartiality*. Oxford: Clarendon Press.

Barry, B. (2001). *Culture and equality*. Cambridge: Polity.

Beveridge, W. (1943). *The pillars of security*. New York, NY: MacMillan.

Blake, R. (2009). *From rights to needs: A history of family allowances in Canada*. Vancouver: University of British Columbia Press.
Brennan, S. (2014). The goods of childhood and children's rights. In F. Baylis & C. Macleod (Eds.), *Family making: Contemporary ethical challenges* (pp. 29–48). Oxford: Oxford University Press.
Brighouse, H. (1995). Neutrality, publicity, and state funding of the arts. *Philosophy and Public Affairs*, 24, 35–63.
Brighouse, H. (2004). *Justice*. Cambridge: Polity.
Brighouse, H. (2006). *On education*. London: Routledge.
Brighouse, H., & Swift, A. (2003). Defending liberalism in education theory. *Journal of Education Policy, 18*, 355–373.
Brighouse, H., & Swift, A. (2006). Parents' rights and the value of the family. *Ethics, 117*, 1.
Brighouse, H., & Swift, A. (2014). *Family values: The ethics of parent-child relationships*. Princeton, NJ: Princeton University Press.
Callan, E. (2002). Autonomy, child-rearing and good lives. In D. Archand & C. Macleod (Eds.), *The moral and political status of children* (pp. 118–141). Oxford: Oxford University Press.
Clayton, M. (2006). *Justice and legitimacy in upbringing*. Oxford: Oxford University Press.
Cohen, G. A. (2008). *Rescuing justice and equality*. Cambridge, MA: Harvard University Press.
Conly, S. (2012). *Against Autonomy: Justifying Coercive Paternalism*. Cambridge: Cambridge University Press.
Donaldson, S. & Kymlicka, W. (2013). *Zoopolis: A Political Theory of Animal Rights*. Oxford: Oxford University Press.
Dworkin, R. (1978). Liberalism. In S. Hampshire (Ed.), *Public and private morality* (pp. 113–143). Cambridge: Cambridge University Press.
Dworkin, R. (1985). Can a liberal state support art? In *A matter of principle* (pp. 221–236). Cambridge, MA: Harvard University Press.
Dworkin, R. (2000). *Sovereign virtue*. Cambridge, MA: Harvard University Press.
Firestone, S. (1970). *The dialectic of sex: The case for feminist revolution*. New York, NY: Morrow.
Frank, R. (1999). *Luxury fever: Money and happiness in an era of excess*. Princeton, NJ: Prineton University Press.
Galston, W. (1989). Civic education in the liberal state. In N. Rosenblum (Ed.), *Liberalism and the moral life* (pp. 89–102). Cambridge, MA: Harvard University Press.
Gheaus, A. (2015). The 'intrinsic goods of childhood' and the just society. In A. Bagattini & C. Macleod (Eds.), *The nature of children's well-being: theory and practice* (pp. 35–52). Dordrecht: Springer.
Gilbert, D. (2007). *Stumbling on happiness*. New York, NY: Knopf.
Griffin, J. (1986). *Wellbeing*. Oxford: Oxford University Press.
Gutman, A. (1987). *Democratic education*. Princeton, NJ: Princeton University Press.
Hurka, T. (1996). *Perfectionism*. Oxford: Oxford University Press.
Kymlicka, W. (1995). *Multicultural citizenship*. Oxford: Oxford University Press.
Kymlicka, W. (2002). *Contemporary political philosophy*. Oxford: Oxford University Press.
Layard, R. (2005). *Happiness: Lessons from a new science*. London: Penguin.
Lecce, S. (2003). Contractualism and liberal neutrality: A defence. *Political Studies, 51*, 524–541.
Lecce, S. (2008). *Against perfectionism: Defending liberal neutrality*. Toronto: University of Toronto Press.
Levinson, M. (1999). *The demands of liberal education*. Oxford: Oxford University Press.

Macedo, S. (2015). *Just married: Same-sex couples, monogamy, and the future of marriage*. Princeton: Princeton University Press.

Macleod, C. (2002). Liberal equality and the affective family. In D. Archard & C. Macleod (Eds.), *The moral and political status of children* (pp. 212–230). Oxford: Oxford University Press.

Marx, K. (1978). Economic and philosophic manuscripts of 1844. In R. C. Tucker (Ed.), *Marx-Engels reader* (pp.66–125). New York, NY: Norton.

Mill, J. S. (1966). On liberty. In J. M. Robson (Ed.), *John Stuart Mill: A Selection of his works* (pp. 1–148). Toronto: Macmillan.

Mulhall, S., & Swift, A. (1997). *Liberals and communitarians*. Oxford: Blackwell.

Nettle, D. (2006). *Happiness: The science behind your smile*. Oxford: Oxford University Press.

Nussbaum, M. (2000). *Women and human development*. Cambridge: Cambridge University Press.

Offer, A. (2006). *The challenge of affluence: Self-control and wellbeing in the United States and Britain Since 1950*. Oxford: Oxford University Press.

Parfit, D. (2000). Equality or priority? In M. Clayton & A. Williams (Eds.), *The ideal of equality* (pp. 81–125). London: Macmillan.

Patten, A. (2014). *Equal recognition: The moral foundation of minority rights*. Princeton, NJ: Princeton University Press.

Quong, J. (2011). *Liberalism without perfection*. Oxford: Oxford University Press.

Rawls, J. (1971). *A theory of justice*. Cambridge, MA: Harvard University Press.

Rawls, J. (1993). *Political liberalism*. New York, NY: Columbia University Press.

Sher, G. (1997). *Beyond neutrality*. Cambridge: Cambridge University Press.

Smith, R. (2009). The long slide to happiness. In R. Cigman & A. Davis (Eds.), *New Philosophies of Learning*. Oxford: Wiley-Blackwell.

Sunstein, C. (2014). *Why nudge?*. New Haven, CT: Yale University Press.

Swift, A. (2006). *Political philosophy: A beginners' guide for students and politicians*. Cambridge: Polity.

Sypnowich, C. (2003). Equality: From liberalism to Marxism (and back again). *Political Studies Review, 1*, 233–243.

Sypnowich, C. (2014). A new approach to equality. In R. Merrill & D. Weinstock (Eds.), Political neutrality: A re-evaluation (pp. 178–209). London: Palgrave Macmillan.

Sypnowich, C. (2017). *Equality renewed: Justice, flourishing and the egalitarian ideal*. London: Routledge.

Victor, P. A. (2008). *Managing without growth: Slower by design, not disaster*. Cheltenham: Edward Elgar.

Waldren, M. S. (2013). Why liberal neutralists should accept educational neutrality. *Ethical Theory and Moral Practice, 16*, 71–83.

On the permissibility of shaping children's values

Andrée-Anne Cormier

ABSTRACT
According to Harry Brighouse and Adam Swift, parents have a limited and conditional moral right to deliberately shape their children's values and interests in light of their own particular comprehensive convictions. Their view contrasts with Matthew Clayton's account of legitimate childrearing, according to which it is always impermissible for parents to seek to pass on their particular convictions to their children or, more generally, to 'enroll' them into their conception of the good, since this violates a requirement of respect for children's independence. This paper offers a novel defense of Brighouse and Swift's position that at least some forms of comprehensive enrollment are permissible. First, I argue that the claim that there is a duty to respect the independence of very young children is problematic. Then, drawing on Brighouse and Swift's account of familial relationship goods, I argue that seeking to pass on comprehensive values or beliefs to one's children is actually compatible with proper respect for their independence, as Clayton understands it.

Introduction

This paper examines the issue of whether it is morally acceptable for parents to deliberately shape their children's values or ends, according to their own particular convictions. In their important book, *Family Values: The Ethics of Parent-Child Relationships* (2014), Harry Brighouse and Adam Swift argue that parents have a limited moral right to intentionally shape their children's particular values and interests in light of their own – provided that this is conducive to meeting children's most fundamental interests, which crucially include the development of their capacities for autonomy and for a sense of justice. Their view contrasts with Matthew Clayton's well-known account of legitimate childrearing (2006, 2012, 2015), according to which it is always impermissible for parents to deliberately seek to instill in their children particular beliefs on so-called 'comprehensive' issues, such as 'religion, occupation, lifestyle, and sexuality' (Clayton, 2012, p. 353).

Contrary to Brighouse and Swift, Clayton believes that parents have no right (not even a limited and conditional right) to deliberately encourage their children to endorse specific controversial beliefs about what activities are worth pursuing, what is valuable, how to live or how to conceive the world. More generally, he thinks that it is always morally wrong for parents to 'comprehensively enroll' their children into a conception of the good or worldview, such as any religious view. This implies, for instance, that it is impermissible for parents 'to baptize their child or include her within religious ceremonies' (Clayton, 2012, p. 362).[1]

One important source of disagreement between Brighouse and Swift, on the one hand, and Clayton, on the other, concerns the issue of how to understand parents' duties regarding children's autonomy. Clayton believes that parents have a duty to facilitate the development of their children's autonomy, understood as an 'end-state' or as an 'achievement,' that is, as the possession and exercise of a capacity to rationally form, revise, and pursue some particular goals, in a context characterized by a sufficiently rich set of alternatives. But parents also have a separate duty to respect their children's autonomy as 'independence' (henceforth, simply 'independence'), where the latter is a matter of not having others decide for oneself which ends to pursue. Brighouse and Swift seem to oppose the idea that there is a duty to respect children's independence (2014, p. 170), at least as Clayton understands it. However, in their book they do not present in detail their reasons for their skepticism. Yet, the issue is important. In fact, according to Clayton, the duty to respect children's independence provides the strongest reason for rejecting comprehensive enrollment. If so, it also provides a direct challenge to Brighouse and Swift's position.

My main goal in this paper is to take up Clayton's important challenge and propose a novel defense of the view that at least some forms of comprehensive enrollment are morally permissible. In particular, my aim is to provide new support for Brighouse and Swift's position by showing, first, that the claim that there is a duty to respect the independence of very young children is questionable and, second, by arguing that the requirement to respect children's independence, as Clayton understands it, does not in any case support his conclusion that comprehensive enrollment is always impermissible. Rather, it supports the view that some forms of comprehensive enrollment, namely, those that promote *autonomy-as-achievement*, are, all other things equal, morally permissible.[2]

The paper is structured as follows. I will start by examining, and rejecting, Clayton's first argument against comprehensive enrollment, i.e. the argument from the cost of rejection. According to it, comprehensive enrollment is impermissible because it makes children's later revision or abandonment of their parents' conception of the good emotionally too costly and, as such, undermines autonomy. I will argue that neither of the two most plausible ways of conceiving the relationship between the emotional costs of revision and autonomy supports the conclusion that *all* forms of comprehensive enrollment are impermissible. I will then reconstruct, and raise doubts about, Clayton's second argument against comprehensive enrollment, which appeals to his idea of respect for independence. According to it, comprehensive enrollment is impermissible because, insofar as parents cannot reasonably expect their children to *retrospectively consent* to being enrolled into a particular conception of the good upon reaching adulthood, it violates children's independence. I will argue that Clayton's defense of his principle of retrospective consent is unconvincing, since it overlooks a morally significant difference between two ways in which an individual can lack a 'capacity for autonomy.' I will consider different possible understandings of the principle of retrospective consent. Drawing on Brighouse and Swift's account of familial relationship goods, I will show that at least some forms of comprehensive enrollment can actually pass what seems to be the most plausible test of respect for children's independence, namely, what I call the 'anti-perfectionist test of retrospective consent.' Finally, I will consider, and rebut, an important objection concerning the aim of parents who seek to shape their children's values.

Preliminaries

Before proceeding to a critical assessment of Clayton's view, it is worth presenting the three main premises around which the liberal debate over comprehensive enrollment is centered. These premises explain why many liberal philosophers writing on familial justice, like Clayton as well as Brighouse and Swift, think that comprehensive enrollment raises difficult ethical questions.

The first, and most basic, premise is that children have an independent moral status. They are not their parents' property and have fundamental interests of their own. In fact, some of their interests are weighty enough to ground the attribution of moral rights to them as well as corresponding duties on the part of others. The second premise is that the parent-child relationship is non-voluntary and coercive for children. The latter cannot escape or consent to being in a relationship with their parents. This relationship is thus authoritative and coercive in nature. This explains why the deliberate shaping of children's values can be seen as *prima facie* more morally troubling than adult-to-adult 'value-shaping' (or 'value-influencing') – to use Brighouse and Swift's expressions. The reason is that, unlike most adults, children do not typically have the capacity to select or leave their intimate relationships and to reflect autonomously on the influence that others exercise on them. In addition, shaping children's values is a special kind of exercise of authority over them, namely, one that has a profound influence on their lives. This is in fact the third premise framing the debate.[3] Values are special because they are identity-defining. They govern people's ends. They are part of what makes persons who they are. So, shaping a child's values appears to be much more significant, morally speaking, than other exercises of parental authority, such as, e.g. the choice of making one's child eat pasta rather than rice for dinner.[4]

Given that children are independent moral beings, and that shaping their values potentially implies shaping how they will aspire to live, in a coercive manner and without their autonomous consent, the question arises as to whether, why, and to what extent, comprehensive enrollment is morally permissible. For his part, Clayton maintains that comprehensive enrollment is never permissible. In the next sections, I will examine, and reject, the two main arguments offered by Clayton in favor of this conclusion: the argument from the cost of rejection and the argument from retrospective consent.

The argument from the cost of rejection

Clayton's first argument states that comprehensive enrollment renders the rational revision or abandonment of one's parents' conception of the good emotionally too costly, in a way that undermines one's ability to rationally pursue alternative goals (Clayton, 2006, pp. 106–107).[5] Clayton does not deny that it can be psychologically difficult to reject one's parents' conception of the good also for individuals who have not been 'enrolled into it.' This is because the ideals and practices that a child is exposed to during childhood always have significant 'emotional grip' – perhaps especially when they are her parents' identify-defining beliefs. However, Clayton believes that comprehensive enrollment exacerbates the emotional costs of revising or rejecting one's parents' beliefs, up to the point of undermining one's ability to opt for a different conception of the good. To be sure, Clayton recognizes that comprehensive enrollment is compatible with the development of the capacities required for autonomy-as-achievement. Still, he thinks that comprehensive enrollment generates psychological costs of rejection so high as to impair one's disposition and aptitude to effectively endorse values, and pursue aims, different from those of one's parents, in accordance with one's own rational judgment. In other words, he thinks that comprehensive enrollment undermines one's ability to exercise autonomy, by adopting and pursuing goals that one rationally finds more plausible and attractive.[6]

In order to properly assess this argument, it is useful to begin with the following question. How exactly should we envisage the relationship between autonomy and the emotional cost of rejection? The argument seems to point to two possibilities. The first is that, above a certain threshold of emotional cost, a person is unable to exercise autonomy and counts thereby as non-autonomous. Let us call this 'the threshold view.' The second possibility is that the higher the emotional cost, the less is a person able to exercise autonomy and, as such, the less autonomous she is. Let us call this 'the degree view.'

Consider the threshold view. In order for the claim that comprehensive enrollment is always impermissible to hold, it must be the case that *all* instances of comprehensive enrollment impose such a high emotional cost of rejection on the child that she becomes unable to exercise her autonomy. However, this seems implausible. In fact, Clayton himself seems to recognize this, for he simply talks about the psychological difficulty of rejecting one's parents' beliefs as a result of comprehensively enrollment. Clayton also explicitly recognizes that comprehensively enrolling a child is compatible with educating her 'such that later in life she can autonomously decide to continue with or reject the religion into which she has been enrolled' (Clayton, 2015, p. 130). This is enough to conclude that, despite the fact that comprehensive enrollment may generate high rejection costs, it is not the case, even by Clayton's own lights, that such costs are always higher than the threshold required to prevent the future adult from exercising autonomy.

Consider now the degree view. To the extent that the ability to exercise autonomy is not linked to a specific level of emotional cost, this view seems to avoid the objection raised against the threshold view. However, the argument based on the degree view presents two other problems. First, it does not seem to be the case that comprehensive enrollment always generates higher emotional costs of rejection and, thereby, a lower degree of autonomy, than non-comprehensive educational approaches. Indeed, as pointed out by Brighouse and Swift (2014, pp. 170–171), as well as by Cameron (2012, pp. 350–351), people enrolled into conceptions of the good that attribute great value to autonomy, such as liberal Anglicanism or secular humanist views, are not especially likely to find it very difficult to revise or even abandon their parents' comprehensive beliefs. Similarly, it is far from clear that abandoning one's parents' beliefs is always less emotionally costly for those who were not enrolled into a particular conception of the good. Children who were not enrolled into a conception of the good may still be very aware of what their parents' deepest convictions are, and may still fear disappointing their parents by not endorsing those convictions.

To illustrate this point, imagine two parents who attribute great value to art and artistic creativity as part of their conception of the good. The first parent deliberately tries to instill this view in her child, while the second does not (i.e. she tries to remain as neutral as possible about the value of art and artistic creativity in making educational decisions for her child). Suppose that both children eventually form the belief that art and artistic creativity have very little value, and that 'art-oriented' careers and goals are not worth pursuing. Is there reason to think that taking this stance will inevitably be emotionally more costly for the first child? The answer seems negative. A parent who refrains from comprehensively enrolling her child does not necessarily care less about what her child comes to believe. In fact, she might be as disposed as the first parent (e.g. because of her character or her especially deep identification with certain ideals) to be disappointed, and to let this transpire, if her child comes to endorse different values than her own (or assign them very different weight). Again, if that is true, it suggests that the emotional cost of rejection is determined by factors not necessarily related to comprehensive enrollment per se.

The second problem with Clayton's argument is that it is not clear whether the degree view itself is a plausible view of the relationship between emotional cost and autonomy. For one, the degree view seems to imply that not incurring any emotional cost when rejecting previously held views is a sufficient condition for a person to count as maximally autonomous. However, this claim is questionable. Indeed, as suggested above, abandoning a previously held conception of the good may be emotionally difficult for anyone, even for fully autonomous persons, since conceptions of the good are identify-defining. In fact, that it is emotionally difficult for a person to abandon her parents' conception of the good may in some cases indicate that that person was genuinely and autonomously committed to it.

The upshot is the following. Whether Clayton adopts the threshold view or the degree view of the relation between emotional cost and autonomy, his conclusion that comprehensive enrollment is always impermissible does not hold. Thus, Clayton's first argument is unpersuasive.

The argument from retrospective consent

The second, and most important, argument offered by Clayton – the argument from retrospective consent – holds that comprehensive enrollment is always impermissible because it is intrinsically autonomy-violating. This argument is best understood in light of Clayton's distinction between autonomy-as-achievement and autonomy-as-independence (2012).[7] Recall that, according to the former, an autonomous person is one who possesses and exercises a capacity to rationally form, revise, and pursue some particular goals, in a context characterized by a sufficiently rich set of options. According to the latter, autonomy is a matter of not having others decide for oneself which ends to pursue, of not being forced or manipulated into pursuing some particular goals. As we have seen, Clayton thinks that individuals have an interest not just in setting goals for themselves, but also in not having others setting goals for them. That is, they have an interest not just in autonomy-as-achievement, but also in independence.

The risk of violating independence is high when decisions are taken for individuals who are unable to decide for themselves. In order to assess whether independence is violated in such cases, Clayton proposes a test that appeals to the idea of retrospective consent whereby an individual's independence is violated if she cannot reasonably be expected to retrospectively consent to (or at least not reject)[8] the decision that is made on her behalf. We can call this Clayton's 'principle of retrospective consent.' This principle is at the heart of Clayton's second argument against comprehensive enrollment.

Here is my reconstruction of the overall argument.[9] The starting point is the claim that (1) there is a duty to respect each person's independence. Clayton holds that (2) the independence of a person who is unable to make autonomous decisions (in the achievement sense) is violated if she cannot reasonably be expected to retrospectively consent to the decision that is made for her. From (1) and (2), it follows that (3) the person in a position to decide for another who is unable to make autonomous decisions has a duty to decide for the latter person in light of reasonable expectations about her retrospective consent. Clayton claims that (4) when a person in a position to decide does not know the content of the other person's beliefs, she cannot reasonably expect that other person to retrospectively consent to being treated according to a particular conception of the good because she may turn out not to endorse that particular conception of the good. Thus, (5) if an individual decides to treat a person according to a particular conception of the good, she violates that person's independence.

According to Clayton, this line of thought applies directly to children. In fact, even though children are currently unable to make autonomous decisions, they will be able to do so in the future and thereby to retrospectively consent to or dissent from how they were treated. From (1), it follows that (1′) there is a duty to respect children's independence. From (2), it follows that (2′) children's independence is violated if they cannot reasonably be expected to retrospectively consent to the decisions that are made for them. From (3), it follows that (3′) parents, who are in a position to decide for their children, have a duty to decide for them according to principles or ideals to which they can expect their children to retrospectively consent. From (4), it follows that (4′) since parents do not know the content of their children's future beliefs, they cannot reasonably expect them to retrospectively consent to being comprehensively enrolled. Hence, (5′) when parents comprehensively enroll their children, they violate their independence. Therefore, from (1′) and (5′), it follows that (6′) the comprehensive enrollment of children is impermissible.

Clayton's argument by analogy

Clayton's most recent and most detailed attempt to defend the principle of retrospective consent when applied to children is by means of analogies designed to convince the reader that choosing for a non-autonomous child or infant, in a way to which she cannot reasonably be expected to retrospectively consent, does indeed violate her independence.[10] He gives the following example:

Skin Graft plus Nose Job: Betty, who is an unknown visitor, is rendered unconscious by an accident and is having a skin graft to restore the damaged skin on her face. The doctor also sees that Betty's nose might be a more attractive shape and so fixes that as well (Clayton, 2012, p. 357).

Clayton suggests that Betty's situation is analogous to a child's situation in two important respects. The first is that Betty is unable to make autonomous decisions. The second is that the doctor does not know Betty's informed preferences, nor her conception of the good. The first point is true of children (or at least infants); the second of parents who have authority over them. According to Clayton, this example is important because, in Betty's case, we would clearly say that the doctor has done something wrong by deciding to fix her nose. More specifically, Clayton thinks that this wrong is captured by the idea of retrospective consent. His idea is that if respect for someone's independence requires getting her consent, which is surely highly plausible, respect for the independence of someone who is unable to make autonomous decisions requires deciding for her according to ideals, norms or principles that will most likely elicit her retrospective consent. In Betty's case, as Clayton puts it: 'When she returns to consciousness, we are almost certain that Betty will thank the surgeon for the skin graft, but far less confident that she will endorse the nose job' (Clayton, 2012, p. 357). Importantly, if Betty's situation is relevantly analogous to a child's situation, then this example shows that a child's independence can similarly be violated when her parents decide for her according to ideals that she cannot reasonably be expected to retrospectively consent to.

I share the intuition that Betty's independence has been violated. I am also willing to accept the connection that Clayton establishes between independence and retrospective consent in this case. However, this does not commit us to accepting the view that young (or at least very young) children's independence is similarly violated when their parents decide for them without taking into account the retrospective consent requirement. The reason is that there is a morally significant disanalogy between Betty and a young child, which renders the application of the principle of retrospective consent more doubtful in the case of young children.

Let us start by presenting the disanalogy. Both Betty and a typical young child are unable to make autonomous decisions. In a sense, we can then say that both are unable to exercise autonomy (in the achievement sense). However, the sense in which this is true for each of them is different. Betty has an already developed capacity for autonomy, whose exercise is simply temporarily blocked. In normal circumstances, e.g. when she is not asleep, or in a coma, or sedated, she is capable of forming, revising, and pursuing a conception the good. By contrast, a young child lacks a well-developed capacity for autonomy. Although she might have the potential to develop such a capacity – if she has the necessary genetic or cognitive resources and if she receives an adequate education, in the adequate context or environment, etc. – she is currently incapable of forming, revising, and pursuing a conception the good. The difference between Betty and the child is thus that Betty is unable to make autonomous decisions just because her already developed capacity to exercise autonomy is temporarily hindered, whereas the child is unable to make autonomous decisions because as a child, she lacks the capacity for autonomy altogether.

I believe that this disanalogy is morally significant. The reason is that an individual who is temporarily unable to exercise her capacity for autonomy has a special interest in being treated in a way that she could retrospectively consent to, which an individual who does not possess such a capacity does not have.

The interest in question is an interest in living one's life and being treated by others in accordance with, and in a way that respects, one's convictions and preferences about how to live and about what is valuable. Such an interest is thus grounded in the individual's possession of a (minimally developed) capacity to form, revise, and pursue a conception of the good. Hence, it is an interest that an individual who lacks such a capacity altogether does not possess. To put things differently, we can say that the interest in not having others setting goals for oneself, which is at the heart of the conception of autonomy-as-independence, is fundamentally grounded in the possession – at least to a minimal degree – of a capacity for autonomy in the achievement sense. It is an interest that one possesses because one has particular goals to begin with, and is capable (to a minimum degree) of rationally pursuing and identifying with them.[11]

This has important implications for the present case. For a start, it shows that young children or at least infants are not akin, from a moral point of view, to sleeping or unconscious people. Most importantly, the previous considerations support the conclusion that, although there may be a duty to respect the independence of temporarily unconscious individuals – a duty that requires us to make decisions for them that they can be expected to retrospectively consent to – there may be no corresponding duty to respect the independence of non-autonomous babies and young children. If so, unless the existence of such a duty can be vindicated in some other way, Clayton's argument by analogy fails to uphold the use of his principle of retrospective consent as a moral constraint on our treatment of very young children.[12] If so, then Clayton's claim that practices such as, for example, the baptism of infants are always impermissible loses some plausibility.[13]

Comprehensive enrollment and the shaping of retrospective consent

Suppose, for the sake of argument, that parents do have a duty to respect their young children's independence. There is another important issue that is worth considering. It concerns the exact formulation and implications of Clayton's test of respect for independence. As presented above, the principle of retrospective consent allows us to determine when an individual's independence is violated, by specifying a sufficient condition for independence violation. Ideally, however, a complete test of respect for independence should also allow us to determine when an individual's independence is not violated. How can this desideratum be satisfied?

A natural option – to which Clayton himself hints at times[14] – consists in formulating the principle of retrospective consent in a bi-conditional, rather than a conditional, form. Accordingly, we can say that an individual's independence is violated if, and only if, the person deciding for her cannot reasonably expect that the individual will retrospectively consent to the decisions that are made for her, while she is unable to autonomously decide for herself. This is equivalent to saying that having reasonable expectations about an individual's retrospective consent is both necessary and sufficient for respecting her independence. Let us call this '*the principle of retrospective consent**.' At first sight, this principle seems quite plausible. In what follows, however, I will argue that, when it is applied to children, it generates counter-intuitive implications.[15]

As a starting point, consider premise (4') of Clayton's argument. As we have seen, this premise states that parents cannot reasonably expect their children to retrospectively consent to having been raised according to their conception of the good, since they do not know whether their children will actually endorse their conception of the good. This premise can be challenged. The main problem with it is that it fails to take into account the fact that retrospective consent can be shaped by education. If parents do a good job at comprehensively enrolling their children into their conception of the good, it is indeed highly likely that the latter will later consent to how they were educated. So, if parents can reasonably be confident that they will be successful at transmitting their conception of the good to their children by enrolling them into it, then they can *also* reasonably expect that their children will retrospectively consent to their enrollment.

In addition to challenging premise (4'), these considerations put some pressure on the principle of retrospective consent*. When applied to children, the principle holds that if children can reasonably be expected to retrospectively consent to the decisions that are made for them, then their independence is not violated. As we have seen, however, parents may form reasonable expectations about their children's retrospective consent by influencing consent through comprehensive enrollment. The principle of retrospective consent* thus entails that in this case children's independence is not violated. This conclusion seems counter-intuitive. If so, Clayton faces a dilemma. If he agrees that the previous conclusion is intuitively incorrect, then he must admit that the principle of retrospective consent* is not a good test of respect for independence. On the other hand, if he is unwilling to abandon the principle of retrospective consent*, then he must grant that comprehensive enrollment is, after all and all other things equal, morally permissible, since it passes the test of respect for independence.[16]

An anti-perfectionist argument in favor of comprehensive enrollment

A possible response to the previous dilemma consists in revising the principle of retrospective consent* by combining it with a more demanding and idealized account of what counts as a 'reasonable expectation.' Clayton's earlier work, which draws explicitly on Rawls's conception of political legitimacy, offers a promising suggestion. Clayton maintains that parents ought to educate their children in ways that could be justified on the basis of public (or what I will call *anti-perfectionist*) reasons[17] in the Rawlsian sense, that is, reasons that any reasonable person could accept no matter what conception of the good she endorses.[18] Simply put, in negative terms, these are reasons that do not appeal to, or presuppose, the truth of any particular conception of the good or controversial philosophical, moral or religious ideal. In light of this, Clayton may say that parents' expectations about their children's retrospective consent count as reasonable if, and only if, there exists an anti-perfectionist justification in support of their educational decisions.

Let us call the resulting principle 'the anti-perfectionist principle of retrospective consent*.' This principle implies that, in order to determine whether comprehensive enrollment respects children's independence, we must determine whether there exists an anti-perfectionist justification in favor of comprehensive enrollment, which can appropriately ground parents' expectations about their children's retrospective consent.[19] Clayton believes that no such justification exists. In this section, I will defend the opposite view. My argument is built around Brighouse and Swift's account of the ethics of shaping children's values, which I will now sketch in its main lines.

According to Brighouse and Swift, in order for children's most fundamental developmental interests to best be met – including their interests in developing the capacities required for autonomy (-as-achievement) and for a sense of justice, as well as for regulating their emotions and connecting with others – they need to be engaged in an intimate and loving relationship with at least one parent. Brighouse and Swift further argue that an intimate and loving relationship unavoidably involves some degree of what they call 'value-shaping.' The reason is that some value-shaping is an inevitable by-product of value-sharing. In turn, value-sharing is required by two important ingredients of a successful loving and intimate parent-child relationship: spontaneity and authenticity.

Spontaneity and authenticity are crucial for a good parent-child relationship for two main reasons. The first is that children need close and loving role models to meet their developmental needs. Parents who make educational decisions 'robotically,' without spontaneity and authenticity, are unlikely to inspire identification. The second, and perhaps most important, reason is that parents can hardly experience their relationship with their children as a source of joy and fulfillment without 'being themselves' in the relationship. In fact, children benefit most from their relationship with their parents when their parents perceive it as rewarding. Thus, it is in children's own interest that their parents experience the relationship with them as a source of meaning and joy (Brighouse & Swift, 2014, pp. 153–155).

Brighouse and Swift are aware that value-*shaping* is not always an unintended effect of value-*sharing*. Some parents deliberately seek to shape their children's values in light of their own particular convictions. In other words, they seek to comprehensively enroll them into their conception of the good. Brighouse and Swift hold, however, that some deliberate value-shaping is crucial to intimacy because the sustainability and depth of any intimate relationship demand that the parties share some common interests and values. According to them, this supports a limited parental right to deliberately shape their children's values in light of their own, for two reasons. First, in early years, only parents can supply the values to be shared in the relationship, since young children do not yet have values of their own. Second, children's emerging value-commitments are typically much more plastic than those of adults. So, parents can legitimately give some priority to their own values in exercising their authority – even when children begin to develop their own values and interests.[20]

Although Brighouse and Swift appear to be skeptical about the idea that there is a parental duty to respect children's independence – at least as Clayton understands it – I believe that their account can be used to show precisely that, under certain conditions, comprehensive enrollment does pass the test of respect for independence, as defined by the anti-perfectionist principle of retrospective consent*. Indeed, Brighouse and Swift's account supports the following line of thought. Children's most fundamental developmental interests, including their interest in developing a capacity for autonomy, are best met when they are engaged in an intimate and loving relationship with at least one parent. As we have seen, an intimate and loving relationship requires some deliberate value-shaping. So, children's most fundamental developmental interests are best met when they are engaged in a parent-child relationship that involves some deliberate value-shaping. If this is true, however, there exists an anti-perfectionist justification for deliberate value-shaping. The reason is that any reasonable person could recognize, no matter what particular conception of the good she endorses, that she, as a child, had a fundamental interest in fully developing her capacity to adopt, pursue and revise a conception of the good.[21] Yet, if the development of such a capacity is tied, in the way just described, to some deliberate parental value-shaping, then that person can also reasonably be expected to retrospectively consent to having been subject to such deliberate value-shaping, no matter what conception of the good she endorses.

One objection against this argument concerns its scope. One may argue that the previous argument vindicates, at most, some very mild forms of deliberate value-shaping, but not more 'global' forms of comprehensive enrollment, such as enrollment into a particular religion. The underlying thought is that comprehensive enrollment of this kind is never necessary for the development of a good, intimate and loving, parent–child relationship. It is perhaps very costly for some parents to refrain from engaging in it. However, by itself, this does not give a reason to the child to later consent to how she was educated.

Three things can be said in response. First, even if we granted this objection, the previous argument would still reach some significant conclusions, considering that Clayton deems to be impermissible any parental action deliberately aimed at passing on specific convictions on issues like sexuality, work, life-style, or religion. Second, arguably, in particular cases, some parental efforts to comprehensively enroll their children into their conception of the good may in fact be necessary for developing a close parent-child relationship. For some parents – perhaps especially religiously committed parents – comprehensively enrolling their children, e.g. by baptizing them, bringing them to church and teaching them the value of things like spirituality, or family ties, or love, as they understand it in light of their religious view, may not only be an important source of fulfillment and joy, but also a key and indispensible element of what it means for them to be authentic in building a connection with their children. Third, it is in any case not clear that comprehensive enrollment must be necessary for developing a close parent-child relationship, in order to elicit children's retrospective consent. More specifically, it is not unreasonable to think that a child may retrospectively consent to comprehensive enrolment when, and because, the latter facilitates, at least to some non-negligible degree, the development of an intimate relationship with her parents, one that serves her own fundamental developmental interests.

If these considerations are on the right track, then they offer a direct confutation of Clayton's argument. In particular, they show that, if the anti-perfectionist principle of retrospective consent* is the correct way to determine whether or not parents' educational decisions respect their children's independence, then at least some forms of comprehensive enrollment are, all other things equal, morally permissible. Having said this, it is worth emphasizing that the previous considerations vindicate only a conditional and limited moral permission for parents to engage in comprehensive enrollment – or to deliberately seek to shape their children's values in light of their own. The latter is permissible only when, and insofar as, it favors the development of parent–child intimacy in a way that serves children's 'neutral' developmental interests, including their interest in developing, and exercising, a capacity for autonomy-as-achievement. This suggests that, all other things equal, it is impermissible for parents to comprehensively enroll their children in ways that either undermine their future capacity to reject those values, *or* completely disregard their children's emerging capacity for autonomy during childhood.

The problem of parents' intentions

In the previous section, I argued that at least some limited forms of comprehensive enrollment are morally permissible, since they can be justified by appeal to anti-perfectionist considerations. However, Clayton might not be persuaded. According to him, violations of independence involve a specific intention, namely, the intention to set another individual's goals. An adequate test of respect for independence should thus focus not just on whether there exists an anti-perfectionist justification in favor of the decision that are made for an individual, but also on whether the person deciding for that individual has appropriate aims.

Based on this, Clayton may present the following objection. Whenever parents comprehensively enroll their children into their conception of the good, they have the intention to deliberately shape their children's values. But the intention to deliberately shape children's values necessarily involves the intention to set children's ends or to decide for them which goals they should pursue. In Clayton's own terms, when parents are 'motivated by adherence to a particular comprehensive view,' then, no matter the content of their comprehensive view, their conduct 'involves the assertion of a right to determine one's child's goals' (Clayton, 2012, p. 363). If this is true, then comprehensive enrollment violates children's independence.

This objection against comprehensive enrollment is particularly strong. It implies that comprehensive enrollment is morally objectionable even when it is conducive to meeting children's fundamental developmental interests. Indeed, insofar as parents have the intention to set their children's ends, then the latter cannot reasonably be expected to consent to their parents' decisions, for these decisions evidence a lack of recognition of their independence. In what follows, however, I will argue that this objection can be resisted. More specifically, I will suggest that deliberately seeking to shape children's values does not necessarily involve the assertion of a right to fix their ends.

My starting point is the claim that it is possible for 'comprehensively motivated' parents – those who make parenting decisions in light of their particular comprehensive (e.g. religious) convictions – to be genuinely and strongly committed to the development of their children's autonomy-as-achievement. As a matter of fact, many comprehensively motivated parents (religious and non-religious) do assign great value to autonomy, for their own particular comprehensive reasons. Yet, if parents are genuinely committed to promoting the development of their children's autonomy, then they are also committed to the idea that their children should be able to decide for themselves which goals to pursue, as they develop their ability to do that. But if they believe that their children should decide for themselves, then they are also committed to recognizing that they have no right to fix their ends for them.[22]

It is true that when a parent baptizes her child, or brings her to church, or teaches her to appreciate art, she intends to increase the likelihood that her child will come to understand and appreciate the values associated with, respectively, a religious faith and artwork. But when such a parent assigns great value to autonomy and is genuinely committed to the development of her child's autonomy, then, while seeking to shape her child's values, she remains open to (and in fact cultivates) the prospect that her child might endorse a different set of values. If this is true, then a comprehensively motivated parent can have the intention (or aim) to shape her child's values without also having the intention to set her ends or to decide for her.

These considerations allow us to clarify a related aspect of Clayton's position. In his earlier work, he distinguishes the attitude of actively seeking to make it the case that one's child comes to endorse certain values or ends (i.e. the attitude which I referred to as the intention to deliberately shape children's values) from the attitude of hoping that this will be the case.[23] He thinks that the former is morally impermissible, but the latter is not. As we have seen, however, Clayton fails to recognize that seeking to impart comprehensive convictions does not necessarily involve deciding for one's child which ends she should pursue. Given this, Clayton also fails to recognize that a parent's intention to shape her child's values *can* sometimes be combined with the hope that her child will come to endorse certain values. In fact, this combination is precisely the one that best characterizes the attitudes of a comprehensively motivated parent who greatly values autonomy and is deliberately committed to developing her child's autonomy.

This suggests that, contrary to what Clayton maintains, the attitude of seeking to impart comprehensive convictions in one's child is not morally objectionable in itself. Such an attitude is impermissible when it is combined with the intention to set one's child's ends; but it is permissible when it is combined just with the hope that one's child will adopt one's values as her ends. This is, of course, simply another way to say that autonomy-friendly forms of comprehensive enrollment are, all other things equal, morally permissible.

Conclusion

In this paper, I argued that Clayton's arguments against comprehensive enrollment are vulnerable to some serious objections. I also argued that, under certain conditions, some forms of comprehensive enrollment are morally permissible by (what I take to be) Clayton's own lights. More specifically, drawing on Brighouse and Swift's account, I showed that comprehensive enrollment can pass Clayton's retrospective consent test when it is conducive to a good, loving, spontaneous and authentic, parent–child relationship, which serves the developmental interests of the child and, in particular, the development of her capacity for autonomy.

Notes

1. For simplicity, in what follows I will mainly talk about 'comprehensive enrolment'. I will use this term to refer to the idea of seeking to impart in children a more or less comprehensive set of particular controversial commitments or beliefs about the value of certain activities and aims.
2. I will not take position on the further question of whether parents have a (conditional and limited) *right* to comprehensively enroll their children into their conception of the good.
3. Clayton (2006) explicitly builds his arguments against children's comprehensive enrollment on the second and the third premises. Brighouse and Swift (2014) agree with these claims (although not with Clayton's conclusion). In my view,

these are not simply premises in Clayton's arguments; rather, they are, together with (1), the basic assumptions framing the debate.

4. Unless, of course, the choice of the meal is value-laden.
5. Clayton calls this the 'instrumental argument'. See Clayton, 2006, p. 106.
6. For this reason, I believe that the argument is best understood as an argument from autonomy-as-achievement.
7. See Clayton, 2012, pp. 359–361.
8. For simplicity, from now on I will omit this qualification.
9. My reconstruction is mostly based on Clayton's, 2012 paper, in which he specifies and defends his view in response to Christina Cameron's (2012) objections.
10. See Clayton, 2012.
11. For a similar line of thought, see Bou-Habib & Olsaretti, 2015, p. 23.
12. Notice that my argument does *not* imply that it is permissible for parents to ask doctors to perform nose jobs (or other similar surgeries) on infants unable to give their informed consent, in order to fix their body according to their esthetic preferences or religious beliefs. Indeed, there are many reasons for thinking that interventions of this type are morally problematic. For one, they are very invasive, medically risky and painful, which implies that they are very likely to have a significant negative impact on the child's current and future wellbeing. They also violate bodily integrity, which – we may think – children have an interest in even *before* they begin to develop a capacity for autonomy. In addition, in certain cases such interventions may also undermine the child's *future* autonomy, for instance by limiting her options in a morally unacceptable way (e.g. the option of enjoying sex in the case of female circumcision). These are just a few considerations showing that the absence of an obligation to treat infants and young children according to the principle of retrospective consent does not have obvious counter-intuitive implications. These considerations also show that Clayton's nose job example is over-determined.
13. This remains compatible with the idea – which Brighouse and Swift endorse – that parents have a duty not just to promote the development of their child's *future* autonomy, but also to respect their children's *emerging* autonomous commitments and interests. This is different, however, from saying that they have a duty to respect the independence of non-autonomous children, as Bou-Habib and Olsaretti (2015) have also noted.
14. See Clayton, 2012, pp. 257–258.
15. I thank Jonathan Quong for suggesting to me the line of thought developed in this section.
16. A possible reply to this objection consists in saying that, in the previous case, it is not children's independence that is violated, but the demands of autonomy-as-achievement. According to this line of thought, the fact that parents can reasonably expect their children to retrospectively consent to their enrollment is indeed *sufficient* to ensure that their independence has been respected. Yet, by comprehensively enrolling their children in such a way as to significantly increase the likelihood of their retrospective consent, parents fail to ensure the proper development of their children's autonomy-as-achievement. This implies that, while the principle of retrospective consent* offers a good test of respect for independence, it needs to be complemented with a test concerning respect for autonomy-as-achievement. (For a similar reply, see Bou-Habib & Olsaretti, 2015, fn. 10, pp. 22–23.).

    It is not clear, however, that this reply succeeds. For a start, it does not seem to offer a correct diagnosis of the case in question. According to Clayton's characterization, manipulating children's goals is a paradigmatic instance of independence violation, not of autonomy-as-achievement violation. In addition, the reply seems to have a limited scope. Indeed, it does not seem impossible for parents to increase the likelihood of children's future consent through comprehensive enrollment, while, at the same time, satisfying the demands of autonomy-as-achievement. For instance, parents might educate their children in a way that significantly increases the cost of rejection of their conception of the good, while making sure they also develop their capacity for autonomy to a sufficient degree. (Notice that this remains compatible with the considerations put forward in the section on the cost of rejection.)

17. Clayton calls this the 'public reason restriction'. See Clayton, 2006, p. 93.
18. A reasonable person, according to Rawls (1993, pp. 49–60), is a person who is committed to the idea of society as a fair system of cooperation between free and equal persons and who recognizes the existence of reasonable disagreement about the good.
19. If an anti-perfectionist justification exists, then children can reasonably be expected to consent to the decisions that are made for them *independently of the conception of the good that they presently endorse*, since an anti-perfectionist justification is one that any reasonable person could accept.
20. Yet, as suggested in fn. 13, parents are *also* under a duty to eventually try and adapt to their children's own evolving values and interests by engaging with them in a respectful and open-minded way (see Brighouse & Swift, 2014, p. 156).
21. In the same way, she could recognize that she had an interest in developing a sense of justice and an ability to regulate her emotions and to emotionally connect with others. These interests are not tied to any particular conception of the good.
22. It seems reasonable to guess that many comprehensively motivated parents would refuse to give their children a 'value-determining pill' which would make it the case – as Brighouse and Swift (2014, p. 162) imagine it – that their children end up endorsing their conception of the good. I take this to support my claim.
23. Clayton writes: 'We must distinguish between an individual's *hope* that someone else comes to affirm her atheism, say, and her seeking to make it true (or more likely) that he does' (Clayton, 2006, p. 115).

Acknowledgements

I am especially grateful to Jonathan Quong and Mauro Rossi for very useful suggestions and feedback on previous versions of the paper. I would also like to thank Harry Brighouse, Christine Tappolet, Sarah Stroud, Christine Sypnowich, Kristin Voigt, Daniel Weinstock, and Danielle Zwarthoed for helpful comments and discussions on issues addressed in the paper.

Disclosure statement

No potential conflict of interest was reported by the author.

Funding

This project has received funding from the European Research Council (ERC) under the European Union's Horizon 2020 Research and Innovation programme [Grant Agreement Number: 648610].

References

Brighouse, H., & Swift, A. (2014). *Family values: The ethics of parent-child relationships*. Princeton, NJ: Princeton University Press.

Bou-Habib, P., & Olsaretti, S. (2015). Autonomy and children's well-being. In A. Bagattini & C. Macleod (Eds.), *The nature of children's well-being. Theory and practice* (pp. 15–34). Dordrecht: Springer.

Cameron, C. (2012). Debate: Clayton on comprehensive enrolment. *Journal of Political Philosophy, 20*(3), 341–352.

Clayton, M. (2006). *Justice and legitimacy in upbringing*. Oxford: Oxford University Press.

Clayton, M. (2012). Debate: The case against the comprehensive enrolment of children. *Journal of Political Philosophy, 20*(3), 353–364.

Clayton, M. (2015). Anti-perfectionist childrearing. In A. Bagattini & C. Macleod (Eds.), *The nature of children's well-being. Theory and practice* (pp. 123–140). Dordrecht: Springer.

Rawls, J. (1993). *Political Liberalism* (Expanded ed.). New York, NY: Columbia Classics in Philosophy.

For a political philosophy of parent–child relationships

Daniel Weinstock

ABSTRACT
In *Family Values*, Harry Brighouse and Adam Swift argue that parents should, in sharing values with their children and in conferring advantage upon them, act in ways that realize the intimacy that lies at the core of the value of family life. In their view, they should prescind from autonomy-inhibiting activities not required by the need to maintain intimacy. I argue that while this standard is sufficient to distinguish between permissible and impermissible practices of advantage conferral, it does not provide us with a perspicuous standard with which to distinguish among activities of value-sharing. This is because the difference between permissible and impermissible forms of value-sharing is adverbial rather than categorical. I argue moreover that even if we were to solve this problem, we would end up with another problem, to do with the unattractive nature of the state activities that would have to be set up in order to police family life. I conclude that the problem of how to enforce the child's right to autonomous upbringing is best thought of as a political one. Schools, rather than the home, are the appropriate site for the development of autonomy, and the state appropriately regulates schools to ensure that they achieve this end.

Introduction

Family Values is the most systematic and philosophically sophisticated account that we possess of the ethics of parent–child relationships. It will be a touchstone in the burgeoning literature on familial ethics for years to come. It is both sensitive and tough-minded. It has been written by two philosophers who have clearly drawn from their own experiences of what makes for successful relationships between parents and their children. It is filled with passages that make not only philosophical but also emotional sense. But it does not shirk before the philosophical difficulties that are given rise to by this puzzling but central relationship. Parent–child relationships are filled with paradox and puzzle, many of them emanating from the fact that what seems so natural from the point of view of parents, namely the sharing of values and traditions and the conferral of advantage, is deeply problematic from the point of view of an even moderately impartialist normative theory.

In this essay, I want to focus on one of the puzzles that lies at the heart of the argument of *Family Values*. The puzzle has to do with the transmission by parents to their children of their most cherished commitments. Arguably, parents could not parent well were they to prescind in parenting from transmitting values[1] to their children. However, the transmission of values risks undercutting the child's ability to form and adopt her own values. If parents have an obligation to contribute to the development of their children's autonomy, there would seem to be a tension, verging on contradiction, among parents' obligations. They both ought to attempt to transmit their values, because in so doing they parent well, and ought not, because in so doing they detract from the autonomy of their children.

I will argue that Harry Brighouse and Adam Swift never completely solve the tension that they rightly uncover in their account of familial ethics. My main point will be that their inability to do so is due to the fact that theirs is, at the end of the day, as the subtitle of their book indicates, an *ethics* of parent–child relationships. What we need in order to overcome the tension among duties is a *political philosophy* of such relationships, one that broadens the focus that Brighouse and Swift bring to the study of childhood in at least two ways. First, such a political philosophy would attend to a greater degree than the authors do to the full range of socially controllable causal factors that go into the upbringing of children. Second, it would pay greater attention to the role of the state in ensuring that the rights of children to the conditions for autonomy, which are made vulnerable in the parent–child relationship, are upheld.

I will proceed in the following manner. First, I will briefly summarize what I take to be Brighouse and Swift's central argument concerning the tension that arises when considering the role of parents in transmitting values to their children, and what their proposed solution to that tension is. I will then proceed to show that it is both indeterminate and unenforceable. That is, parents seeking guidance in how, exactly, to balance their obligation to attend to the autonomy of their children, while at the same time parenting them according to their values, will come away from the book without a clear set of principles with which to negotiate the tension. But even if we are able to fill in the blanks somewhat, it turns out that they are unenforceable, or rather that they are enforceable only at the cost of ascribing excessive powers to the state. If the rights of children depend solely upon the success of parents in instantiating these principles, or in being coerced to do so by the state, then we are presented with a very unattractive dilemma. Finally, I will propose a solution to this dilemma, one that distributes the obligation to uphold the right of children to a number of agents, and in particular, to schools.

Can familial intimacy and the autonomy of the child be reconciled?

Should parents be permitted to transmit their values to their children? From a certain point of view, this question may seem pointless, a philosopher's question in the pejorative sense of that term. *Of course*, one might want to say, parents both can and should transmit their values to their children. After all, parenting is a value-laden affair, and what other values than their own might parents appeal to in raising their children? Moreover, it would seem, no one is harmed when parents draw from their values in going about the business of raising their children.

This naïve take on the issue is however disturbed by the fact that while it may at first blush seem clear that parents should have the right to parent their children on the basis of their values, it is also clear that children should be raised in a manner that fosters their autonomy. And there may be a number of things that parents do in the course of transmitting their values to their children that fall foul of this requirement.

One way out of this dilemma has been attempted by Matthew Clayton, in his much-discussed book *Justice and Legitimacy in Upbringing* (Clayton, 2006). Clayton argues, in effect, that since parents represent from the point of view of their children a kind of mini-state, in that they wield power over their children from which children cannot exempt themselves, it follows that they should behave toward their children just as liberal states ought to do, evincing neutrality with respect to their conceptions of the good in the way in which they wield their power, and devoting themselves to the development of the autonomy of children above all other developmental goals.

As Brighouse and Swift argue, however, this account of parenting as entirely constrained by norms of liberal public reason is 'too costly' in terms of other relationship goods, ones that give parent–child relationship their independent value (Brighouse & Swift, 2014, p. 178). Brighouse and Swift's view is built around the idea that the parent–child relationship is distinctive. Its value cannot be reduced or accounted for in terms of other kinds of relationships, such as that of friendship or of romantic attachment. At the center of that relationship is a kind of intimacy that is different from the intimacies that adults share with other adults. According to Brighouse and Swift (2014, p. 91), 'the parent is bound by his fiduciary responsibilities for the child's emotional development to try to be spontaneous and authentic a good deal of the time, both because the child needs to see this modeled and because the child needs to be in a loving relationship with a real person'. Treating one's children as if one were merely a public official would severely detract from the ability to parent according to this conception of intimacy. This is because part of what it means to be intimate and authentic with one's children is to share one's enthusiasms with them, to enact the values one believes in, to share with them in the practices (religious or not) that one finds meaningful, and so on. To prescind from doing so when around one's children would introduce an emotional barrier between parents and children that would take away significantly from the value of their relationship.

Clayton is not insensitive to the value of intimacy within a parent–child relationship, but he thinks that intimacy can be made compatible with the avoidance by parents of 'enrolling' their children in their comprehensive conceptions. He writes that 'children may witness and take pleasure in their parents' comprehensive accomplishments without being schooled in the virtues and practices of the comprehensive conceptions or affirming its value' (Clayton, 2006, p. 171).

Clayton's argument here is grounded in a very counterintuitive distinction, which is that one can as a parent display one's values in a manner that reflects all of the importance one ascribes to them, without in so doing transmitting one's belief in that value to one's children, so that they remain in a 'witnessing' relationship to parental enthusiasms, and avoid the risk of becoming excessively affected by them. Indeed, it seems tolerably clear that when one displays or enacts one's values authentically, one transmits something of these values, even if one's intention is not to transmit them, much less to detract from one's child's autonomy in so doing. It is an unavoidable side-effect of a parent behaving authentically and spontaneously in the manner required by Brighouse and Swift's view (one that as we have seen is shared by Clayton, to the extent that he does not deny the importance of intimacy to the parent–child relationship) that she risk making those values more attractive, and therefore, more eligible, to her child.

But just as Clayton is sensitive to the value of intimacy in a parent–child relationship, so are Brighouse and Swift alive to the importance of raising children in a manner that does not detract from the development of their autonomy. They write that 'on our account of the duty of care, the parent is obliged to do what she can to ensure that her child has the capacity [...] to decide for herself how she is to live her life' (Brighouse & Swift, 2014, p. 157). Thus, Clayton on the one hand, and Brighouse and Swift on the other, are in substantial agreement as to the ethical challenge that parents must face: they must parent in accordance with their values while ensuring that in so doing they do not impermissibly detract from the autonomy of their children, but rather contribute to that development. Where they disagree has to do with their respective proposed solutions to this quandary. We have seen that Clayton's solution (that parents display their values, while maintaining the emotional and epistemic status of their children as mere witnesses to that display) is implausible. Do Brighouse and Swift fare better?

In considering whether or not parents have the right to confer advantage upon their children, Brighouse and Swift hit on the following criterion: there are certain activities, such as the reading of bedtime stories, that conduce to the quality of the familial relationship. Now, it turns out that children who have stories read to them by their parents fare better in all kinds of ways than do children who are deprived of bedtime stories. But because the intimacy that comes from bedtime story rituals is central to the achievement of healthy parent–child relationships, it follows that it is allowable, even though it can demonstrably be shown to give rise to inequalities among children. Sending children to expensive private schools in order for them to acquire a competitive advantage over their peers is on their view not allowable, because it confers advantage without being necessary to the achievement of familial goods.

It is more difficult, as Brighouse and Swift acknowledge, to bring this criterion to bear upon allowable and impermissible ways of shaping values. This is because, 'the kinds of interaction that lead to the shaping of children's values by parents are integral to family life, on our conception of it, because they are central to a successful parent–child relationship' (Brighouse & Swift, 2014, p. 153). Thus, as opposed to the case of the conferral of advantage, one cannot in the case of the shaping of values distinguish particular *kinds of actions* from which one must prescind. Rather, the creation of intimate familial relations is made compatible with the fostering of the autonomy of children through the *manner* in which one engages in (potentially) value-shaping activities. Thus, one must avoid shaping one's children's values through brainwashing techniques (an easy case); but one must also restrain oneself from 'exerting emotional pressure' (Brighouse & Swift, 2014, p. 173). To put it in terms of a slogan, the difference between permissible and impermissible kinds of parenting is categorical in the area of advantage conferral, and adverbial in the case of value-shaping. On Brighouse and Swift's account (2014, p. 155; my emphasis),

> as long as [...] deliberate shaping of values is needed for a close relationship between parent and child, and as long as it is done *in a way* that is consistent with the duty to develop the child's capacity for autonomy, then, on our account, parents have a right to engage in it.

Can parents avoid 'emotional pressure'?

From this summary of Brighouse and Swift's argument with respect to the shaping by parents of their children's values, it should be clear just how difficult it is to provide parents with a clear set of action-guiding prescriptions as to how to go about the business of parenting their children in a manner that both conduces to the intimacy of the parent–child relationship and is protective of the child's development of her autonomy. Now, there are clearly some ways of parenting that fall far foul of the line separating permissible and impermissible forms of value-shaping. Brainwashing, threats of violence, extreme emotional blackmail, shunning and ostracism – these and other ways of attempting to inculcate values in children are clearly morally odious.

But that we are able to make these determinations does not speak to the power of the criterion developed by Brighouse and Swift. First, the case against these parenting strategies is overdetermined. It is not just a concern with the autonomy of children that makes us reject them. Basic kindness and a concern for the emotional well-being of children, to cite only these two considerations, also speak decisively against these harmful parenting practices.

Second, it is unclear whether these kinds of impermissible forms of parenting are actually ways in which parents seek to get children to share their values. Rather, they seem to be ways in which to get children to behave in certain ways rather than others. Now, it may be the case that for certain parents, shaping behavior, rather than belief about value, is all that matters. But the interesting cases, and the ones that a theory such as Brighouse and Swift's should have something to say about, are ones in which parents try to get their children to endorse the same values as them in ways that are detrimental to their autonomy. And it is not clear that their view provides them with a way of addressing those cases.

Consider the restriction that they place against parents being allowed to 'exert emotional pressure' on their children to get them to share their values. The exertion of emotional pressure encompasses a very broad range of kinds of behavior and attitude, some of which should actually be countenanced or even encouraged by Brighouse and Swift, given their view of healthy, intimate familial relationships. Indeed, a parent who in the presence of her children displays enthusiasm and passion in engaging in the activities that she finds valuable is, by this very fact, exerting emotional pressure upon her children. If her relationship with her children is healthy, then they will tend to be emotionally disposed to find pleasing the things their parents take pleasure in. When parents act on this disposition, whether they do so intentionally or not, they are exercising emotional pressure. And yet they are doing something that would seem to be called for by the theory of familial intimacy under discussion.

Now, parents can also engage in far less subtle forms of emotional manipulation. They can threaten to withdraw affection when their children fail to conform to their value wishes, or perhaps even worse, they can insidiously inflect their emotional responses in ways that make their children know that they are not pleased with the values on the basis of which their children have chosen to act. These shadings of emotional response can be all but imperceptible to everyone but those who are involved in the relationship, and who are alive to the manner in which an action or a reaction that might seem innocuous to the outsider 'counts' as a mark of disapproval.

Perhaps, the criterion we are looking for in distinguishing permissible from impermissible emotional pressure has to do with intentionality. The parent who acts enthusiastically on her values, and who moreover does so in a manner that suggests to her child that she will be disappointed were the child not to follow suit, does nothing wrong, though she does clearly exert emotional pressure. When the parent acts on her child's emotions in a way that is not simply the spontaneous manifestation of her beliefs, but is designed to affect the child's decision-making process, or even more subtly, her emotional disposition with respect to her parent's values, then she acts impermissibly.

I am not sure that this moral distinction can be upheld, however, or if it can, it requires yet more layers of distinctions and nuance. Imagine a parent who has always professed a set of political values. Imagine that these values have an impact on the way she leads her life on a daily basis – on the way in which she interacts her others, on the consumer choices she makes, and so on. Imagine moreover that her belief in these values is so deep as to color not just her actions, but the emotional tenor with which she carries out these actions.

Now imagine that her child rejects these values. One can imagine a parent expressing her disappointment. Indeed, not to do so would lead us to question the seriousness with which she held these values in the first place. A conscientious parent will take care to reassure her child that her disappointment does not detract from her love for her child. Perhaps arguing about politics can become one of the intimacy-creating activities that parent and child engage in. But it would be a lot to ask of a parent that she not display some disappointment. In so doing, she would be manifesting a reactive attitude that has, among its many other functions, the function of attempting to affect the attitudes of the agent with whom she disagrees.[2] Now, clearly, the parent needs to take care in the manner in which this disapproval is expressed. I think, however, that it would be incompatible with our view that parents have deep commitments, and that they display these commitments through their actions to their children, that they not, in virtue of the depth of their commitment, express disappointment when their children choose to reject these values and exercise gentle emotional pressure caused by the hope that the child might come to change her mind.

The example just provided is not decisive, but it invites the thought that the line separating permissible from impermissible emotional pressure is a subtle one, one that it would be very difficult to formulate in terms of an action-guiding principle. And if this case generalizes to other ways in which parents act in a value-shaping way, it follows that parents looking to Brighouse and Swift's criterion – that they can engage in value-shaping activities to the degree that these are necessary for the creation of intimacy, but only if they do so in a way that is compatible with their children's autonomy – will be left in the dark when hard cases arise, and where certain kinds of parenting are not ruled out by a plethora of values, of which a concern with the autonomy of their children is just one.

It might be objected[3] that I have just formulated precisely the kind of action-guiding criterion that I have claimed is impossible on Brighouse and Swift's account. To wit, I have claimed that the conscientious parent will in expressing her disappointment make plain that it does not detract from her love for her child. Is this criterion not enough to guide the action of parents with intensely felt values who are nonetheless committed not to exert undue emotional pressure upon their children?

I would argue that it is not. First, the attitude that must be struck by parents seeking to strike a middle ground between disappointment and reassurance is, as I have shown, a very subtle one, and it is unrealistic to expect that even well-intentioned parents will be able to achieve it. Action-guiding principles must guide action not just among perfectly wise parents, but among 'good enough' parents as well.

This points back to a second, deeper point. Emotional pressure is not to be understood on the model of a scale, with disapproval on one side of the scale being negated by emotional reassurance on the other. Though this is not a philosophical point, I believe it is plausible to suggest that emotional pressure survives even as steps are taken to attempt to counteract it. Parents must prescind from manifesting disappointment rather than doing other things to leaven that disappointment with approval, if they are to avoid exercising undue emotional pressure.

Bringing the state (back) in

We have arrived at a very unhappy place, philosophically speaking. We have recognized, with Brighouse and Swift, that there are ways in which parents transmit their enthusiasms and values that are more or less compatible with the autonomy of their children, and that they should avoid those ways of engaging in value-shaping that are incompatible with autonomy. Yet we have also seen, though a brief engagement with the notion of 'emotional pressure', that it is difficult to formulate an action-guiding principle neatly distinguishing permissible and impermissible modalities of emotional pressure.

Things are in fact worse still. For even if there were some way of distinguishing (within the class of ways in which to pass on values the impermissibility of which is determined by considerations of kindness or concern with emotional well-being only indirectly related to the preservation of autonomy) between permissible and impermissible ways of passing on values, we would then be left with a cruel dilemma: either enforcement of the relevant principle falls to the state such as we presently find it in most liberal democracies, with the result that the distinction will go unenforced, or we provide the state with the means with which to enforce the distinction, in which case we end up with a state that violates liberal democratic strictures that we have good reasons to want to uphold.

Let me begin this part of the argument by making what I hope will be a fairly uncontroversial observation. The moral right of children to be raised in ways that are not incompatible with their being able to exercise autonomy in later life is an important one, one that warrants being guaranteed through the coercive apparatus of the state. The interests that lie at the basis of the obligation that both Clayton, and Brighouse and Swift recognize on the part of parents to bring up their children in ways that conduce, or that are at the very least not incompatible with the development of the child's capacity for autonomy, are of sufficient weight, in other words, not to make their realization simply a function of the ability and the disposition of parents to uphold the relevant principles, but rather to entrust that realization to state institutions. Put briefly, there are reasons to make the moral right that children have to an upbringing compatible with autonomy into a legal right.

Though neither Brighouse and Swift nor Clayton develop this point at any great length, there are passages in both of their works that suggest that they too view the realization of the child's right to autonomy as at least in part a matter for state institutions and state officials to take up. Thus, for example, Clayton writes (2006, p. 102; my emphasis) that his argument 'has revolutionary implications for parents *and public authorities*'. And Brighouse and Swift observe (2014, p. 152; my emphasis) that '*the state can do some things* to limit the opportunity for excessive value shaping while respecting the space and discretion that are needed for flourishing parent-child relationships'.

However, if as I have argued, the difference between allowable and impermissible value-shaping is adverbial rather than categorical, that is, if it attached to the manner in which value-shaping is pursued rather than the activities through which it is pursued, then it would seem at first glance as if the right that would protect the child's interest in autonomy is unenforceable, at least under the kinds of liberal-democratic regimes that are being assumed by all of the authors we are considering here. Consider: under present circumstances, the state only intervenes in the way in which parents raise their children in the home under the most extreme of circumstances, that is, when children are subjected to significant physical and emotional neglect and abuse. The state will step in to protect children from their parents, and at the limit to terminate parental rights, only when children are physically hurt by their parents – when they are sexually abused or beaten, or deprived of the necessities of life, or when they are subjected to the worst kinds of psychological and emotional deprivation.

There are many reasons to limit the role of the state to stepping into the home in these extreme kinds of cases. First, the state's role *vis a vis* families in most liberal democracies is premised upon a view of the family that is largely compatible with the view argued for by Brighouse and Swift, namely, that children do best when they are raised by their parents, rather than, say, in state institutions, even when those parents are not perfect (provided of course that they are 'good enough'). Thus, even when parents violate some of the strictures that they would observe were they perfect parents, they are best left undisturbed by the state in their parenting choices.

Second, and relatedly, were the state to broaden the scope of its surveillance and intervention in the home in order to make it responsive and reactive not just to egregious violations of parenting responsibilities, but also to more subtle lapses, it would undermine the conditions under which the kind of intimacy that makes families unique and irreplaceable forms of human relationship is possible. Indeed, it is difficult for parents (or their children) to act with the kind of spontaneity required by intimacy if they feel as if they are constantly being observed, as if they might be subjected to some form of state interference when they fall short of their ethical obligations toward their children. It is unlikely, moreover, that autonomy will be reliably developed if parents are coerced into becoming the agents of that development through the operation of the coercive power of the state.

Third, there is also a concern with the plurality of parenting styles. Once we have excluded the kinds of physical and emotional abuses that the state rightly steps in to prohibit, there can be reasonable disagreement among parents as to how to raise children. Some of these differences can be cultural, others irreducibly individual. The state rightly allows for a degree of reasonable disagreement as to how to parent, once children's most fundamental interests in physical and psychological safety are provided for. Providing the state with the power to interdict styles of parenting that do not seem to conduce to autonomy runs the risk of lapsing into the culturally insensitive practice of interfering with styles of parenting that are neither more nor less compatible with autonomy, simply because they are culturally foreign from the parenting styles of the majority.

If all of this is granted, then we can see the difficulty before us. Even if, contrary to what was argued in the last section, it is possible to distinguish between acceptable and unacceptable ways to shape the values of one's children, the line distinguishing them will be well short of the line that liberal democracies have identified as justifying state action. A child whose parents engage in forms of emotional enforcement of values that, though morally problematic, fall short of the kind of psychological abuse that would warrant state intervention in the life of the family will not be protected by the state, even a state that is committed to the autonomy of children. There is a range of activity in which parents engage which, though falling short of ethical norms, does not rise to the degree of severity that would warrant state intervention.

Now, a theory of upbringing single-mindedly devoted to the development of autonomy might argue that if liberal democracies at present abstain from intervening in the lives of families in cases in which the rights of children to an autonomy-enhancing upbringing are being violated, then so much the worse for liberal democracy. Perhaps, on such a view, the state ought to be more active in defending the rights of children, even when this involves intervening in the home sphere.

There are reasons not to bite that bullet, however, even for a theorist defending the central importance of autonomy in the way in which children are raised. Some of them have already been adverted to. A state that granted itself the permission to act on behalf of the autonomy of children in the intimate sphere of the home would be by this fact undercutting the creation of intimacy, and, most likely, of autonomy-development as well. It would also risk imposing a conception of parenting that enforced the cultural norms of the majority with respect to parenting under the guise of autonomy protection.

But even if we were to put these concerns aside, there are reasons to think that the line distinguishing acceptable from unacceptable kinds of value forming would simply escape the epistemic capacity of states, even ones that had eschewed liberal democratic concerns with excessive surveillance of its citizenry. Remember that the line that we are looking for is one that not only rules out brainwashing, threats and the severest forms of emotional manipulation, but also one that allows us to distinguish between only subtly different forms of emotional pressure on the part of parents. These might not be reflected in easily identifiable actions, but rather in tones of voice, and in gestures and reactions that are in and of themselves innocuous, but acquire significance (and emotional force) only within specific familial contexts. All this is too subtle and fine-grained for even the most surveillance-minded of states to capture. Not only, therefore, would a state devoted to rooting out autonomy-inhibiting parental practices be unattractive from the standpoint of a liberal-democratic ethics. It would also be epistemically inconceivable.

We seem to have reached a kind of impossibility result. We have concluded, it seems, (1) that parents sometimes do act in ways that inhibit the autonomy of their children, that (2) it is important for the state to act in ways that uphold the conditions in which children can develop their capacity for autonomous decision-making, and (3) that there is nothing that the state can do even if it was willing to renounce a liberal-democratic ethics in order to protect children against the autonomy-inhibiting behavior of their parents.

I believe that we can avoid this result, or at least, that we can remove much of its sting. In order to do so, we must remind ourselves of the fact that the family is but one of the institutions that contribute to the upbringing of children. Children also spend a lot of time in schools, as well as in civil society associations such as churches, sports teams, the like. And though, for reasons that we have just discussed, it may be difficult or impossible for the state to ensure that autonomy-promoting conditions exist in the home, it is possible for the state to regulate the other spheres in which children are raised to ensure that the (potentially excessive or heavy-handed) value-shaping that they undergo at the hands of their parents is balanced by autonomy-promotion carried out in other spheres in which they are brought up, and in particular in schools. It is to this solution to our problem that I now turn.

Schooling for autonomy

The work of Brighouse and Swift, but also that of Clayton, has made philosophers of the family and of childhood more sensitive than they had been to the tension that exists, on the one hand, between the conditions for the intimacy of the family, which may involve a not inconsiderable amount of value-shaping as a foreseeable consequence, and the conditions for the development of the autonomy of the child, which may require that children be protected to some degree from the impact of their parents' value-shaping behavior.

Let me begin my proposal for the way out of this tension by pointing out an asymmetry between these normative considerations, both relevant to the manner in which children should be brought up. The asymmetry is this: there is a good inherent to value-shaping when it is carried out by parents that is not matched by autonomy promotion being carried out by parents. In other words, it matters to familial goods that value-shaping occurs within the family. But it does not matter to the value that attaches to autonomy that parents be the agents that bestow it upon their children.

We already have some of the elements needed to establish the first side of this asymmetry to hand. We have already seen that familial intimacy is served when parents are authentic and spontaneous with their children, and that that requires that they act in their presence on the basis of their deepest value commitments and beliefs. The enthusiasm with which they enact their values through their actions may (and very likely will) have an impact on the values of children. What ultimately distinguishes this aspect of the familial bond from an unattractive state paternalism is the fact that the value-sharing that occurs within the family is in the service of an ethically attractive form of human relationship. It is the fact that value-sharing occurs in the context of the construction of a kind of relationship that would be very difficult to construct in the absence of that value-sharing that immunizes it from the kind of critique that would be legitimate in the case of the overly perfectionist state.

Now consider the case of individual autonomy. Does it matter to as great a degree that the autonomous decision-making capacity of children be bestowed upon them by their parents? Obviously, it is *permissible* that parents act in such a way as to promote the autonomy of children. And as we have seen through our discussion of Clayton, and Brighouse and Swift, it is part of an attractive (though unenforceable) parental *ethics* that the value-sharing that occurs within the family be leavened by a commitment to autonomy.

But what if a set of 'good enough' parents were not quite as committed to the autonomy of their children as this ethical view would require of them? What if, instead, the development of autonomy in their children were the result of the operation of another institution? Would it matter for the value of that autonomous decision-making capacity that parents were not themselves its artisans?

I would argue that it would not. There is, as we have seen, something special about the sharing of values within the family that makes it the case that the value transmission that occurs there is permissible, and perhaps even desirable, whereas the transmission of those very same values might rightly come to be seen as invasive and paternalistic were it to result from the operation of another institution, say that of a paternalistic state. But this is not the case for autonomy. Autonomy is a good for children independent of its source. For its justification does not stem from the fact that it is a foreseeable consequence of a range of activities that are necessary for the creation and maintenance of a valuable form of human relationship. Rather, autonomy is a good because of the capacity that it provides children, and the adults they will become, to shield themselves from undue influence and manipulation that others might see fit to visit upon them. That capacity is neither increased not diminished from the fact of having resulted from the operation in the upbringing of the child of one institution rather than another.

If this argument is plausible, it follows that we need not look to just one institution, such as the family, as the sine qua non of the child's autonomy. We need not impose upon it the responsibility of ensuring that the children that are raised within it are raised autonomously. Nor do we need to overtax the state's capacity by requiring that in the name of the autonomy of children it observe the ways in which they are raised by parents in the intimate sphere. Nor need the state stand ready to intervene in that sphere when children are subject to value-shaping which, though it cannot be qualified as brainwashing or rank manipulation, may perhaps be viewed as excessive from the point of view of a parenting ethics that requires of parents that they attend both to ensuring that familial relations are characterized by the requisite degree of intimacy, and that it be a locus for the teaching of autonomous-decision-making. Of course, it may be a *better* form of familial relationship in which both of these objectives are reached. But, as long as there is another institution to which children are subjected, and that has as its main function in the upbringing of children that it contributes to their autonomy, then this juggling act between intimacy and autonomy is not one that we need require of families.

In other work, I have argued that none of the objections that we have canvassed in order to argue against the state intervening in family life in order to promote the autonomy of children applies in the case of schools. State regulation of schools is thus, the best way in which to ensure that among those institutions that participate in the upbringing of children there is one that is devoted to the autonomy of children (Weinstock, 2016). Indeed, whereas there are arguments about the conditions for the intimacy of families that tell against the state intervening in family life to do anything more than protect children against the most egregious negligences and ethical lapses of parents, no such arguments pertain to schools. There is no ideal form of school life that gets distorted by the intervention of the state in the name of the autonomy of children.

What's more, most liberals already accept that the state should be involved in both the funding of schools (to ensure that access to education is equitably distributed) and in their curriculum (to ensure that children are provided with the cognitive tools that they need in order to function as competent adults). Adding a concern with the promotion of autonomy to the tasks that are imparted to schools neither overtaxes the state's epistemic capacity, involves it intruding into a kind of relationship the value of which coexists with great difficulty with state intervention on a systematic scale.

To say that schools can contribute to the task of the development of the autonomy of children is not to say that they should, as it were, teach autonomy. Indeed, autonomy may, like happiness, be a pedagogical objective that is best developed by indirect means (Weinstock, 2004). What is needed in order to achieve the goal of autonomy-promotion is that children acquire the capacity to think critically about the values that contend for their attention and commitment, both those that emanate from their families and those that come from the broader civil society. This can be achieved by having the claims of some conceptions of the good confronted against those of others. Thus, schools need not, in order to achieve the purpose that I have proposed for them here, be Jacobin institutions in which freedom and autonomy are held up and taught as independent values. Rather, what is required of them is that they meet the rather weaker (and more attractive) condition of not simply being vehicles for the values around which the familial domain is organized. Thus, the responsibility placed upon the state in its regulation of schools for the purposes of achieving autonomy is an easily attainable, negative condition.

This conclusion may seem too ambitious for some, and excessively meek for others. On the one hand, some might argue that it is essential to a child's emotional well-being that there not be too much of a conflict between the values that a child learns in school, and those that are imparted in the home. On the other hand, it might seem to some that aiming at autonomy though indirection, by teaching children about other values and forms of life, in the hope (but not the certainty) that this will shake loose the hold of parental values, is insufficiently bold, given the importance of the stake that the development of autonomy in children represents. Clearly, the question of how best to promote autonomy in schools cannot be fully addressed in the context of this short paper. My point has been to argue that schools must be brought into the discussion about how best to promote autonomy, rather than to reach robust conclusions about the conclusions that such a discussion should reach.

Conclusion

I have argued in this paper that the development of autonomy in children is too important to entrust solely to the ethical responsiveness of parents. I have also argued that though there probably is a right way in which to balance the twin objectives of intimacy and autonomy promotion within families, that balance is one that is not amenable to the kind of action-guiding principle to which parents wishing to find the right balance might refer. Finally, I have argued that notwithstanding all of these considerations, the kind of state that would give itself the prerogative and the capacity to enforce such a balance within the intimate sphere of the family would be hugely problematic from the point of view of what we might call 'state ethics'. Better, I argue, to reorient our thinking about the conditions for the development of the autonomy of children politically. The upbringing of children is not the sole responsibility of parents and of the family. It is of too great an importance not to be backed up by the coercive power of the state. And that power, I have argued, is best deployed through the regulation of schools than it is through interventions in the intimate sphere of the family.

Notes

1. I will for the sake of brevity use the term 'values' to refer to a congeries of traditions, passions, commitments, beliefs, that parents pass on to their children while they go about the work of parenting.
2. In writing of reactive attitudes, I am of course making reference to P.F. Strawson's notion, as expounded in 'Freedom and Resentment' (Strawson, 1962).
3. I thank an anonymous reviewer for the Journal, who pressed me to develop this point.

Disclosure statement

No potential conflict of interest was reported by the author.

References

Brighouse, H., & Swift, A. (2014). *Family values. The ethics of parent–child relationships*. Oxford: Oxford University Press.

Clayton, M. (2006). *Justice and legitimacy in upbringing*. Oxford: Oxford University Press.

Strawson, P. F. (1962). Freedom and resentment. *Proceedings of the British Academy, 48*, 1–25.

Weinstock, D. (2004). The problem of civic education in multicultural democracies. In A. Dieckhoff (Ed.), *The politics of belonging nationalism, liberalism, and pluralism* (pp. 107–124). Totowa, NJ: Rowman and Littlefield.

Weinstock, D. (2016). A freedom of religion-based argument for the regulation of religious education. In B. Berger & R. Moon (Eds.), *Religion and the exercise of public authority* (pp. 167–183). Oxford: Hart.

Childhood bads, parenting goods, and the right to procreate

Sarah Hannan and R. J. Leland

ABSTRACT
Harry Brighouse and Adam Swift, together with many other philosophers, think that adults' interests in raising a child can give them a moral right to parent when they will be adequate parents. We consider whether the same interest could give such adults a moral right to procreate, as a means of acquiring a child to raise. We argue that the interest in parenting cannot support a right to procreate, because the features of childhood that make parenting uniquely valuable for adults are bad for children. Adults may have a right to procreate, but they do not have that right due to their interest in a parent–child relationship.

Introduction

In *Family Values: The Ethics of Parent–Child Relationships*, Harry Brighouse and Adam Swift argue that many people have a profound interest in parenting, rooted in the value of the relationship that parents can enjoy with their children. These people's lives would be stripped of unique and important goods if they didn't raise a child. Brighouse and Swift rely on this parental interest to argue that adults who would be adequate parents have a moral right to raise a child, so as to satisfy their relationship-based interests.[1]

Brighouse and Swift don't directly address the ethics of procreation; their concern is the ethics of relationships between parents and existing children, whether biological or adopted.[2] But it's common to believe that procreating is one permissible way – perhaps even the default way – to satisfy the interest in being a parent that Brighouse and Swift's argument draws upon.[3] This is, after all, the way the vast majority of people become parents. It's also impossible for everyone with a strong interest in the parent–child relationship to satisfy their interest without some people making children. Every child who is parented, including adopted children, must be procreated. Even if everyone who procreated but preferred not to parent the resulting children gave those children up to adults with a strong interest in parenting, the demand would likely outstrip the supply. Moreover, the adoption process, at least as it exists in most affluent modern societies, imposes a host of challenges on would-be parents; the process is often expensive, intrusive, and slow.[4] So the unique and powerful interest in parenting that *Family Values* relies on in its case for the right to parent appears, at first glance, to give many adults strong reasons to procreate.[5]

A further thought would move from the claim that adults have strong reasons to procreate in order to parent, to the claim that their interests in parenting suffice to establish a moral right to procreate, provided they would do a good enough job of meeting their children's interests. The interest in procreation might ground a corresponding right – at least when procreating is the only way for competent would-be parents to acquire a child without taking on more costs than they can be expected to in order to satisfy their interest in the parent–child relationship.[6] We call this attempt to derive an entitlement to procreate from an entitlement to parent the 'parental relationship justification' of the right to procreate. Again, Brighouse and Swift don't themselves endorse this argument; they have no official position on the ethics of procreation. But the parental relationship justification of the right to procreate is an interesting and initially plausible extension of their view.

Despite the seeming plausibility of the parental relationship justification, we argue that there is a morally fraught side to adults' interests in parenting, which often goes unacknowledged. This derives from the necessary link between children's subjection to some significantly bad features of childhood, and adults' profound interests in parental relationships with children. The unique relationship goods of parenting outlined by Brighouse and Swift involve helping children to cope with, and eventually overcome, bad-making features of childhood. If children didn't experience these bad features, then parents wouldn't enjoy the unique goods of being a parent.

This dependence of adults' interests in parenting upon children's subjection to the bads of childhood undermines the parental relationship justification of the right to procreate. It does so by undercutting (or perhaps severely attenuating the strength of) the reasons that an adult's relational interest in parenting would otherwise give her to procreate as a means to satisfying that interest. In other words, the interest in the parent–child relationship that would ordinarily speak strongly in favor of the right to procreate fails to do so, because the interest's satisfaction directly requires that children be non-consensually subjected to some very bad states.[7] Since the parental relationship justification of the right to procreate depends on the claim that adults have strong reason to procreate, this result undermines that case.

A few clarifications are needed before moving on. First, the rights to parent and procreate mentioned in the parental relationship justification are moral rights, not legal rights; our focus here is on the interpersonal morality of procreation rather than the law and public policy issues surrounding procreation.[8]

Second, the rights we consider are weighty moral liberties to parent and procreate, paired with entitlements against interference with certain aspects of one's parenting and procreation. So the right to procreate would explain why a person could permissibly procreate, even when her doing so imposed high costs on others.[9] To illustrate, consider that procreating and raising a child results in a massive production of greenhouse gas (likely more significant than any other projects the average person undertakes).[10] Many people believe that the imposition of such costs renders ordinary actions impermissible. However, a right to procreate would explain the commonsense verdict that adults are permitted to procreate despite these consequences, without requiring us to accept that they have rights to impose comparable forms of pollution in service of less significant pursuits. It would also explain why others wrong a would-be procreator if they try to interfere with her procreation.

A final point concerns the paper's target. We consider one explanation of how adults' interests could support a moral right to procreate: Brighouse and Swift's relationship goods account. There are many other ways to defend the right to procreate. For example, procreation might be a way of adding value to the world by creating new persons, honoring religious commandments, or maintaining the existence of a family line or ethnic group. Our argument says nothing about these, or other, justifications, so a right to procreate may well be justified on grounds not examined here.[11]

Our focus on the parental relationship justification may seem narrow, but we think it's worthy of detailed consideration for several reasons. First, it resonates with a common attitude that intentional procreators take toward the decision to create a child. Many parents cite their interest in a special relationship with a child as the reason they decided to procreate. Since the success or failure of the parental relationship justification has implications for the moral evaluation of this decision, it's worthy of sustained consideration. Second, the parental relationship justification is philosophically significant, in light of the prominence and plausibility of Brighouse and Swift's work on parenting. While they don't take a position on the view, it's a natural extension of their work. Moreover, ideas resembling the parental relationship justification figure in several recent discussions of procreation.[12] Finally, we think the parental relationship justification is more promising than many alternate explanations of the right to procreate, including some of those mentioned above. So its failure has significant implications for the prospect of a successful defense of the moral right to procreate.

The remainder of this article proceeds in three parts. Section two discusses the relationship-based interest in being a parent. Section three links this interest to the fact that children experience seriously bad features of childhood. Section four argues that the parental interest doesn't lend strong support to the right to procreate, because the satisfaction of parents' interests depends on and is inextricably tied to their children being subjected to bad states.

Good for parents

Brighouse and Swift believe that 'many, perhaps most, adults need to be involved in an intimate relationship of a particular kind [with a child they parent] in order to have a fully flourishing life' (2014, p. 88). They regard this relationship as contributing uniquely to adults' well-being, such that, for adults who have a profound interest in parenting, other relationships couldn't substitute for the flourishing produced by being a parent.

Brighouse and Swift link the goods of parenting to four special features of the parent–child relationship (2014, pp. 88–91). First, the relationship involves unequal standing between participants: children are especially vulnerable to their caretakers, don't choose to enter the family, and generally lack the power to exit it. Second, children are often unable to look after themselves, so parents must sometimes coerce and manipulate children for their own good. Third, children lack a determinate conception of their own good, such that parents must play a role in shaping what children take to be valuable in life. Fourth, children are primed to spontaneously and unconditionally trust and love their parents.[13]

These features of the parent–child relationship jointly explain why parenting requires a special form of care. Parents have a high-stakes responsibility: shepherding their children through the transition from childhood into self-governance. Their engagement in that role is a source of satisfaction, and it offers some unique opportunities for personal development. More importantly, these features allow parents to enjoy special forms of intimacy and affection with their children, which can be one of the most fulfilling aspects of adults' lives. If parent–child relationships didn't have the four features mentioned above, the mode of care involved would be different, and less significant, at least with respect to the well-being of adults (Brighouse & Swift, 2014, p. 91). Changing these features might deprive parenting of some of its special challenges or joys, such that the interest would not be so weighty; as a result many adults' flourishing wouldn't be so significantly reduced by being denied the opportunity to parent. A change in the parent–child relationship would also blur the lines between parenting and other types of relationships, transforming it into a relationship akin to friendship or other fiduciary relationships, which people could enjoy without having children.

For the remainder of the paper, we assume that Brighouse and Swift's view correctly identifies the interest many adults have in parenting. But what we say about their view generalizes to many other plausible accounts of the interest adults have in parenting. For example, although their views differ in interesting and important ways, Colin Macleod (2010) and Christine Overall (2012) present accounts that share many of the salient features of Brighouse and Swift's account. For our purposes, what's important about all these explanations is that they link the special value of the parent–child relationship for parents to the fact that children are unique beings who need to be cared for and controlled in light of the specific incapacities and challenges they face. We strongly suspect (though we don't consider alternative accounts here) that any attempt to explain the special value of the parent–child relationship will fail to account for its uniqueness or profound importance to adults if it doesn't essentially involve children's asymmetric dependence, vulnerability, and need for parental care and control. Such attempts would fail to show that parenting was non-fungible, thus failing to explain how the interest in the parent–child relationship could support a right to parent or procreate when other relationships are available that satisfy the same interests.

In the next section, we show that it's bad for children to be subject to the incapacities and challenges that establish the special value of parent–child relationships. This puts pressure on the idea that adults' interests in these relationships could support a right to procreate.

Bad for children

Childhood imposes some bad conditions on children. We focus on four bads of childhood: impaired capacity for practical reasoning, need for extensive parental control, profound and asymmetric vulnerability, and lack of an established practical identity. These features are essential to explaining the unique character of the parent–child relationship, and thus the special interest that many adults have in being part of that relationship. But the presence of each of these conditions is significantly bad for children, in the sense that they are significant impediments to children's well-being.[14]

We aren't claiming that the bads of childhood make childhood an overall bad condition for children (as Hannan (in press) does). Nor do we claim that procreation harms or wrongs children, in light of the fact that it exposes them to the bads of childhood. The bads of childhood are features that are regrettable, but, for all we say here, there may be goods of childhood that outweigh the bads, making childhood an overall desirable condition. Children may be able to enjoy certain unique goods that adults cannot (Brighouse and Swift (2014, p. 65) think that sexual innocence is one such good). Alternately, children may have a special propensity to enjoy goods that adults also enjoy, such as special access to the goods of imaginative play (Gheaus, 2015; Macleod, 2015). Our arguments here are compatible with those claims, and with the further claim that the good aspects of being a child are sufficiently weighty to make childhood on the whole good for children. We only claim that some aspects of being a child are significantly bad. These, we go on to show, are the very aspects that generate the unique relationship goods adults can enjoy from parenting.

Impaired practical reasoning

When human agents have aims they want to accomplish, they often set themselves to reasoning about how to accomplish them. Agents also reason about how their aims fit together, with an eye to assuring consistency and coherence in their ends and their plans to achieve those ends. Children are agents that are characteristically bad at this kind of reasoning. They have purposes, but they're not good at determining what means to take to accomplish these purposes. Nor are they good at ensuring that their aims and plans are consistent or coherent.

This inability is partly a result of children's immature capacities for practical reasoning. For example, children are systematically worse than adults at reasoning about what to do when decisions involve probability estimation, as when a decision involves the assessment of risk. The inability also results from children lacking information. They simply haven't been in the world long enough to assemble a body of reliable information, which is necessary to reason effectively. Finally, for the most part, children aren't as good as adults at delaying gratification or managing their emotions. This also prevents them from effectively reasoning and acting in pursuit of their goals.

Children's lack of information and impaired practical reasoning can also lead them to make objectively bad decisions with some frequency. As Brighouse and Swift point out, 'young children explore the world in a way that is largely uninformed about the dangers it presents ... they will consume poisons, walk into busy roads, fall through windows, drown in swimming pools, burn themselves on hot ovens, even if they are warned not to' (2014, p. 63).

These shortcomings suffice to explain why children's impaired practical reasoning is bad for them: it prevents them from getting and doing the things they want (even when these are reasonable things to want), and it leads them to engage in activities that are dangerous. Moreover, children's inability to achieve their ends often leads them to experience considerable frustration and sometimes even anguish, thereby detracting from their well-being.

A more controversial claim concerns whether there's something non-instrumentally bad about being a person – a creature fairly close in its practical capacities to normally functioning adults – that is quite bad at setting ends for herself and determining means to her ends. We're inclined to believe that it's inherently bad for persons to aim for foolish or worthless things, that many of children's aims are for such things, and that this is explained (at least in large part) by their reasoning incapacities. If those thoughts can be successfully made out, then children's impaired practical reasoning could be shown to be bad in its own right, as well as instrumentally bad insofar as it affected children's ability to satisfy their own preferences and desires.

Need for extensive parental control

Children are subject to legitimate parental authority (which can often be permissibly backed by coercion) in many aspects of their lives. For example, when a child only wants to eat unhealthy foods, her parents may, and sometimes must, require her to develop a taste for healthier foods. Good parents' control of their children is often morally unimpeachable. But the fact that children need to be subjected to this control is a regrettable feature of their lives. As with impaired practical reasoning, part of the badness of this need for subjection is a result of children's experience of parental control. Having their actions controlled is often very difficult for children. Some children can find being controlled reassuring, at times. We think the bad experiences are likely to exceed the good, for most children, but we're also more confident than in the case of impaired practical reasoning that this need for control is regrettable apart from the way children experience it.

It's intrinsically bad for a person to be subject to extensive control across a variety of aspects of her life, and parents' control of children is such a kind of extensive control.[15] Systematic subjection to the will of another makes life worse for a being capable of guiding its conduct (even imperfectly) according to judgments about how it ought to act. This result isn't altered by the fact that a considerable degree of subjection is ultimately in children's best interests.

Profound and asymmetric vulnerability

Children are primed to incautiously form attachments: they tend to latch on lovingly to the adults they depend upon (and in some cases to other adults), even when these adults aren't worthy of their love. Children are physically vulnerable to adults as well, since they're smaller and weaker than most adults. Most of the bads of childhood listed above also render them vulnerable to the abuse or neglect of adults (and other children), as well as to non-agential dangers in the world and dangers that result from their own bad decision-making.

Vulnerability is present in, and likely necessary for, a host of valuable relationships, so it may seem strange to regard its presence as a bad. This is especially true in vulnerability-inducing relationships that are consensually entered into on the basis of trust – relationships like engagement in a shared economic venture or romantic partnership, for instance. Children's vulnerability, however, has a number of features that make it unlike the vulnerability present among business or romantic partners, and more like forms of vulnerability that we ordinarily find troubling.

Children's vulnerability to parents is asymmetric. A parent can easily harm her child, but children are generally unable to harm their parents in the same way, or to the same degree, (even if children can have the ability to do hurtful things that prove devastating for their parents). The stakes of children's vulnerability are very high. The harms involved can be grave; children's mental and physical well-being – even their lives – are at stake.[16] Moreover, children aren't normally able to exit their familial relationships to seek out parents who will do a better job of caring for them. If they're to get what they need from adults, most of it will generally have to come from their parents. Social arrangements that make non-parents responsible for a larger share of childcare can mitigate the risks imposed by this vulnerability, exposing children to more styles of caregiving, and ensuring that multiple parties have an eye on the threats to which children are exposed (Gheaus, 2011, pp. 502–505). Conscientious caregivers, parental and otherwise, can also help to protect children from harm. But it's important not to overstate the extent of the protection that adults can offer children. Profound and asymmetric vulnerability is inescapable for children.

When vulnerability eventuates in harm, that vulnerability is clearly bad for children. Children's awareness of their vulnerability can also be a source of distress in their lives, making it a cause of experiential disvalue. But children's profound and asymmetric vulnerability may not seem bad for them in cases where it does not eventuate in harm and they are unaware of it, especially when children are free from harm because conscientious adults protected them. But we think vulnerability is seriously bad, even when it doesn't eventuate in significant harm and children are unaware of it.

One way to appreciate the badness is to recognize that persons have an interest in a modally robust freedom from harm, in addition to their interests in avoiding actual harm. That is to say, they have an interest in being protected from harm in a host of relevantly similar possible scenarios. In everyday contexts, we often discuss this kind of interest as an interest in safety: exposure to significant danger is bad, even in cases where that danger doesn't eventuate. This explains why it's bad for airline passengers to fly on planes that haven't been serviced properly, even if none of the planes actually fails to operate, and the passengers are unaware of the danger. The lack of maintenance exposes the passengers to danger: had things gone slightly differently (had a vital component been marginally less durable, as it might well have been) the plane would have gone down. Children's vulnerability exposes them to a similar kind of danger, even when parents do all we can expect of them to do to guard children against harm. Had things gone differently for those children (had they wandered away in a different direction, for instance), they would have faced significant harm. And we believe their lives are worse in virtue of that danger.

In short, vulnerability that doesn't eventuate in actual harm is nonetheless bad for children because it makes children's protection against harm modally insecure. Good parenting can reduce the insecurity, but there will be a wide array of dangerous scenarios, even under the most safety-promoting rearing. Moreover, there are also compromises that good parents must make between safety for their children and other important goals, such as children's development of their independence. Recall that children's vulnerability is also bad for them to the extent that knowledge of their vulnerability distresses them, and when their vulnerability results in harm.

Lack of an established practical identity

We take impaired practical reasoning, need for parental control, and profound asymmetric vulnerability, to be fairly non-controversial instances of states to which it is bad for a person to be subjected. We now turn to a more controversial candidate for a bad state that is constitutive of childhood: the lack of an established practical identity. There's a sense in which children – especially younger children – often lack an authoritative prospective on what they want. Facts about 'where they stand' as agents aren't fully established, since they haven't developed a stable identity, characterized by various plans and commitments, from which to make decisions about what kinds of projects they want to pursue in the world.

So while a child will commonly want something, this aim is often less robustly her own than it is when she takes it up as an adult. As an adult, she embarks on a project against an established background of other plans and commitments, whereas her aim as a child springs up against a sparser background. As a result, the aim is less fully hers – there's less to say about why she identifies with it. It's also characteristically less stable, since it can be changed without necessarily altering many of her other aims and commitments.[17]

Why think lacking a practical identity is a problem? One explanation is that it prevents children from valuing things deeply in the way adults can. This is bad for children because it that deprives their lives of a core source of meaning.

Children often experience this absence as a problem as well, especially as they mature. They recognize that they need to make their life choices in a way that is coherent and authentic. Without making choices like that, their lives don't go well. Awareness of this fact is one of the core difficulties of later childhood. But childhood involves lacking the capacities necessary to make the choices children are called on to make.

Children's lack of practical identity is less obviously bad for them than the features of childhood discussed above because there seems to be a valuable side to the unsettledness of children's practical identities. Settled plans and projects can be encumbrances as well as sources of value. There are possibilities opened up by the shallowness of children's commitments: they can imagine themselves more readily in wildly incompatible life projects, for instance, in a way that becomes difficult for adults. This kind of imaginative activity *is* valuable. Besides being enjoyable for children, unconstrained imagining helps children to see how things look for others, and to recognize potentially attractive possibilities for themselves. We might also think that children benefit from a special ability to engage in valuable forms of experimentation and play that aren't available to agents with more established identities. This claim can be made more plausible when accompanied by the observation that we characteristically progress from childhood, with a lack of an established practical identity, toward the more established identities characteristic of adulthood. Perhaps a complete life that includes both experiences is better than a life that includes only one, and, if this is right, then the claim that lack of an established practical identity is bad for children is less plausible.

Readers can decide for themselves whether this fourth purported bad of childhood is overall bad for children. We include it because we think it's worthy of consideration, but don't insist on its badness for children, as we do with the previous three.

On the charge that we treat children as little adults

Thus far, we have argued that childhood is significantly bad (at least in some respects) for children, since it involves impaired practical reasoning, the need for extensive parental control, profound and asymmetric vulnerability, and (perhaps) the lack of an established practical identity. One common response to our claims about the bads of childhood is to say that, while they would be bad for adults, they aren't bad for children. Our picture of childhood, the objection goes, is like the depiction of children found in medieval- and renaissance-era paintings, where children are depicted as tiny adults. Critics claim that this isn't what children are like; children are different kinds of creatures from adults, with different interests, such that some things that are bad for adults are not bad for children, and vice versa (Tomlin, in press).

This important objection depends on the fact that what it is for a child's life to go better differs significantly from what it is for an adult's life to go better. In particular, various kinds of agential interference (internal and external) are bad for self-governing adults because such adults have the abilities to govern their own lives, but they aren't bad for children, since they characteristically lack that ability.

We agree that rendering self-governing adults incapable – even temporarily – of governing their lives is worse than creating children who are temporarily incapable of self-governance. For instance, many adults (unlike most children) have autonomously formed preferences that their self-governance continue into the future, coupled with complicated plans they have built their lives around. This makes it especially terrible for them when they lose this capacity for self-governance, or are denied its exercise.

However, we think that having a will – fully formed or otherwise – makes the conditions discussed above bad for children. Children guide their action in light of their assessment of what reasons they have to act. We believe that the conditions enumerated above are very bad ones to be in for creatures that possess a capacity for reasoning practically, however underdeveloped.

Children's experience of these aspects of childhood supports the claim that the conditions discussed above are bad for them. Our claim that these states are bad for children is not made true simply in virtue of children's experiences, but their experiences provide good evidence for the objective badness of the states under consideration. It's possible to be in a bad state, without recognizing as much, and without feeling badly about that state. But when people experience a state as bad, that gives us a strong indication that it actually is bad. And – perhaps with the exception of the lack of an established practical identity – children very regularly experience these states as bad for them. They express their sadness and frustration about their subjection to parental control and their inability to accomplish their purposes on a regular basis. And, especially when their vulnerability is made vivid to them (as when they are harmed or fear that they may be), children often respond with fear or despair. We take these responses to be good evidence for the claim that the bads of childhood are actually bad for children.

The fact that children often experience the states under consideration as bads also plays a role in explaining their badness. After all, frustration, unhappiness, and other negative emotional responses engendered by the bads are conditions which, when regularly experienced, make a life objectively worse than it would otherwise be.

Note also that as children mature they get more and more like adults in terms of their self-governance capacities. Yet there are still intermediate stages where many of the bads of childhood obtain with respect to a child that is part-way to adulthood. If you think the bads would be bad for adults, then there is considerable pressure to regard them as bad for at least some children – namely those who are older, and closer to self-governance, than very young children.

For these reasons we believe that the features of childhood discussed above are bad for children. This can be a difficult conclusion to accept, in part, because it frames adults' relationships to children in a way that appears more problematic than we would often like to acknowledge. It's important to recognize that the bads of childhood are a product of the characteristic features of childhood, not of failed parenting. While different modes of social organization and different choices by parents and third parties affect how bad these states are for children, any feasible mode of procreation and rearing will leave children subjected to impaired practical reasoning, extensive parental control, profound and asymmetric vulnerability, and the lack of an established practical identity.

We have argued that being a child involves occupying a state partly constituted by some seriously bad states. We now consider the how that fact bears on the parental relationship justification of the right to procreate.

Parental Interests and the right to procreate

Parents have a weighty interest in raising children because they're able to enjoy a uniquely valuable kind of relationship with their children. The uniqueness and value of this relationship depend, as Brighouse and Swift have argued, on the fact that children require a special form of care and control. Notice that children require this care and control precisely because they suffer from the bads of childhood. So parents' enjoyment of a special relationship with children is inextricably bound up with children's subjection to the bads of childhood. A child who wasn't an impaired practical reasoner, lacking an established practical identity, needing extensive control, and subject to asymmetrical vulnerability, wouldn't be someone with whom parents could possibly enjoy the special kind of relationship that Brighouse and Swift identify as a major element of many people's flourishing.

This essential dependence of adults' relationship interests on the bads of childhood means that those interests don't speak in favor of a right to procreate, as they would otherwise do. More generally, the benefits enjoyed by care-givers cannot figure in an explanation of why we ought to create scenarios in which someone is in need of their care.

This is obvious in some cases. Suppose that a person would genuinely flourish by nursing a close friend back to health as a result of the intimacy that such care would foster. This in no way speaks in favor of creating a situation in which her friend is ill and in need of care. Similarly, if a person would benefit from helping a romantic partner through a difficult time, this doesn't provide her with good reason to engineer difficulties for her partner. While each caregiver's significant interest in special relationships would ordinarily give strong reason to create a situation in which they enjoy those relationships, this reason is undercut by the fact that the interest essentially requires putting the recipients of care in seriously bad states.

It is less obvious that the benefits to parents cannot figure in the explanation of why they should procreate, because the alternative to subjecting a child to the bads of childhood is that child's non-existence. The relevant contrasts in the other cases aren't like this. Instead, they are scenarios in which a person's friend exists but isn't sick, or a person's partner is around but isn't faced with difficulties.

It's natural to be skeptical of the claim that the bads of childhood undermine the case for the right to procreate for a related reason: children gain access to a host of goods in virtue of existing, and there isn't any way (given the nature of human development and reproduction) for us to create persons without their experiencing the bads of childhood. As a result, procreation can seem to be a way of benefiting children.[18] Even if procreation does benefit the created person, this doesn't vindicate the parental interest justification against our argument. While the child's benefitting may speak in favor of procreation, this wouldn't mean that the would-be parent's relational interest in raising the child speaks in favor of a right to procreate. That interest isn't based on benefiting the child (or at least not solely so); it's an interest in being in a relationship with a creature that's afflicted by the bads of childhood. And a carer's interest of that sort doesn't explain why the carer has a right to bring about the situation in which the delivery of care is possible.

For a further illustration, consider a case that is closer to procreation than those discussed above. Dr. Frankensteen is a lonely scientist living on an island with no other persons. Frankensteen devises a method for creating an artificial life form, Monstra, from inanimate objects. The limits of Frankensteen's scientific powers mean Monstra will inevitably suffer from some serious problems. She'll experience considerable pain and some difficulty getting around. As a result, she'll require considerable care from her maker. On bad days, she'll need Frankensteen to help with her chores and comfort her when the pain gets especially difficult. But if Frankensteen looks after her, Monstra's pain and hardship will gradually decrease, such that she can expect to have typical human abilities after a decade of difficulty. Frankensteen recognizes all this before creating Monstra.

Now consider two different sorts of interests Frankensteen might have in creating Monstra. The first is an interest in friendship. Frankensteen is lonely, and has a strong interest in enjoying an intimate relationship with another being. This interest could be fully satisfied even if Monstra weren't exposed to the bad states she is necessarily afflicted with.

A second possible interest would be in a special form of intimacy that comes from caring for an asymmetrically vulnerable dependent, which Frankensteen would enjoy as a result of creating Monstra and helping her deal with her challenges. This interest fits with a deep commitment to helping Monstra – Frankensteen looks forward to providing that help, and he knows that, with a little luck, Monstra's life will ultimately be a good one, which matters significantly to him. But the bads that Monstra will face play a different role in this interest than they do in the interest in overcoming loneliness. This second interest, unlike the first, wouldn't be satisfied if Frankensteen improved his alchemy and avoided subjecting Monstra to significant difficulties.

Whether Frankensteen has a right to create Monstra will depend on a host of considerations: the appropriateness of creating artificial life, or beings that experience certain levels of pain, for instance. But one consideration that it seems clearly inappropriate to consider in the mix is Frankensteen's interest in caring for someone afflicted by the difficulties Monstra faces, or in being in a special relationship that requires such care. The reason-giving force of that interest is undercut by the fact that its satisfaction requires subjecting Monstra to significant pain and non-consensual dependency. By contrast, the more general relationship interest he has in friendship, which isn't reliant on Monstra's suffering, may well be a relevant consideration. In short, only some relationship interests look relevant to determining whether we have a right to create someone to share a relationship with us.

The kind of parental interest that Brighouse and Swift discuss, and which is also endorsed by some others who present a relationship-based justification of the right to parent, cannot support a right to procreate. This is because these interests are directly reliant on the bads that children face, in the way that Frankensteen's objectionable interest in caregiving was. The parental interest is an interest in a relationship that *necessarily* involves one party being subjected to the bads of childhood. That subjection isn't a mere side effect, as it was when Frankensteen created Monstra to secure a friend. Since the normative force of the caregiver's interest seems to be undercut in the previous cases, we believe the same should be true of this case.

Most people who want to parent have an interest in parenting children from infancy and young childhood. They have an interest in parenting someone who is a poor practical reasoner, who lacks an established practical identify, who needs extensive control, and who is significantly more vulnerable than they are. If you told would-be parents that you could take away these aspects, many would no longer have an interest in parenting, because they could not derive the same special goods from raising such children. The more children come to resemble adults, the less unique our relationships with them become, and the less able they are to contribute specially to our flourishing. Brighouse and Swift (2014, p. 91) acknowledge this in stating that, 'other intimate relationships, where those are consensual on both sides and in which the parties are symmetrically situated, are not adequate substitutes.' They correctly insist that part of what explains the special character of the parent's relation to a child is 'her degree of vulnerability to one's judgments [and] her involuntary dependence' (2014, p. 93). This necessary and direct connection between the parental goods and the bads suffered by children is what undercuts the normative force of adults' interests in procreating in order to parent. Since the parental relationship justification of the right to procreate claims that the normative force of those interests grounds a right to procreate, this undercutting renders the justification unsuccessful.

Our argument depends on the idea that the benefits enjoyed by a caregiver can't figure in an explanation of why the caregiver is entitled to create scenarios in which someone is in need of their care. What would explain that claim? We aren't committed to a particular explanation here, but we find the following line attractive. Asymmetric caring relations between persons can be morally problematic. As persons, all parties involved in these relationships have equal moral status. But relationships where one party depends upon the care of the other, without being able to reciprocate with comparable care of his or her own, can seem at odds with the idea of a relationship between equals. To be sure, these relationships needn't be inegalitarian. They can be compatible with the equality of the parties involved when both parties enter into them by choice, against a background of alternate options. But when an asymmetric caring relationship is imposed without the meaningful consent of both parties, it tends to forcefully threaten the status of the dependent party. One way to overcome this threat is to show how the relationship could be justified to the dependent based on his or her interests alone. If, instead, the creation of the relationship is justified by appeal to the caregiver's interest in a special relationship with the recipient of care, it can seem that the recipient is being treated a means to the caregiver's satisfaction. And this type of treatment is ordinarily incompatible with respecting the dependent's equal status as a person.

This brings us to an interesting potential implication of our argument. The failure of the parental relationship justification may not only mean that parents' interests in a relationship with children fail to ground a right to procreate. It may also indicate that parents who decide to procreate primarily in order to secure the goods of the parent-child relationship behave in a way that reveals a defect of character or motivation. This could be true even if there were other grounds supporting a right to procreate (and hence rendering permissible these parents' procreation). In procreating with the main aim of enjoying the goods of parenting, these people create a situation where someone is exposed to the bads of childhood *so that* they can deliver the care and enjoy the benefits of doing so. This seems to display an objectionable indifference (or unawareness of) the relationship between their own parental interests and the regrettable circumstances of childhood. Since we believe many adults do procreate primarily in order to benefit from parenting, and since the idea of their doing so doesn't initially seem intuitively objectionable to many of us, we find this result interesting and troubling.

One further thought, which we lack the space to explore here, is that adults might have strong reason to adopt in order to satisfy their interest in the parent-child relationship. Adoptive parents' care tends to existing needs. They don't cause a child to suffer from the bads of childhood in the same way that procreative parents do, so adoption escapes the concerns raised in this paper.

Conclusion

We've argued that the relational interest in parenting doesn't speak in favor of a right to procreate. Nothing about this suggests that procreation is morally impermissible – many activities that we don't have a *right* to engage in are sometimes *permissible* to engage in. Our argument is also compatible with the conclusion that there is a right to procreate supported on grounds other than parents' interests in the kind of special relationship identified by Brighouse and Swift. But we take ourselves to have shown that the parental relationship justification fails to support a right to procreate. The goods of parenting depend on the bads of childhood in a way that undercuts the reasons that parents' interests would otherwise give for procreating. Despite initial appearances, parental interests of the kind laid out by Brighouse and Swift are not a promising basis for a right to procreate.

Notes

1. Brighouse and Swift give a dual interest argument for the right to parent, which draws heavily on the interests of children as well as parents. The interests of children explain why only adequate parents have a right to parent on their view. Moreover, Brighouse and Swift set the bar for adequacy quite high in recognition of children's interests. But parents' interests also play a crucial role in establishing the right to parent on their account. One of their aims is to explain why adequate parents would be wronged if their custody of their children was terminated to better satisfy the interests of those children. They claim that the interests of adequate parents are weighty enough to justify retaining custody of their children even when others would do a better job of meeting those children's interests. We focus on the interests of parents here, but what we say is consistent with their complete dual interest view, and its concern for children's interests.
2. In at least two points in *Family Values*, Brighouse and Swift do entertain a connection between procreation and parenting. They say that 'adults who judge themselves unable to love their children may still have reason to procreate – if there are others who want to be parents, who possess and wish to exercise their capacity to love but are not themselves able to procreate' (2014, p. 21). In discussing Christine Overall's work, they state that her 'focus is on procreation, rather than parenting, though of course, in the standard case, people's reasons for wanting to do the former are so that they can get to do the later' (2014, p. 194). These passages suggest they believe parental interests give reasons for procreation, but they don't explicitly endorse this view.
3. Brighouse and Swift now distinguish (appropriately in our view) between the right *to* parent and the rights *of* parents; while the rights of parents are justified by children's interests alone, the right to parent is grounded partially on the interests that adults have in occupying this fiduciary role (2014, p. 54). Our focus here is on adults' interests in the right to parent, and whether these interests also support a right to procreate.
4. The cost excludes many people from adopting, and people are sometimes also excluded because they are single, unmarried, or in same-gender relationships. It's difficult to adopt infants, but many parents' flourishing is linked to raising children from a young age. Moreover, some of the children available to adopt face special challenges, stemming from disabilities or histories of trauma. These challenges may interfere with some would-be parents' flourishing. Many of these challenges are the result of unjust discriminatory features of adoption policies and bionormative cultural views, which we reject. All sorts of people can be good parents, and parental interests can be satisfied by sharing a relationship with biological and adopted children. Nevertheless, even if adoption is an equally valuable or superior form of acquiring a child to raise, one still needs to answer the important question about whether the parental interest in the parent–child relationship can support a right to procreate.
5. Throughout the piece we discuss the rights and interests of 'adults,' 'parents,' and 'would-be parents'. Unless context indicates otherwise, each locution refers to those adults who have an interest in being parents, and whose right to procreate a child is at issue.
6. There are complicated issues concerning the move from interests to rights, which we don't take up here. We simply follow Brighouse and Swift in thinking that there's a plausible move connecting fundamental and widespread interests in parenting to the right to parent (2014, p. 53). They argue that adults' interests in

parenting are weighty enough to give them a right to raise a child, provided doing so doesn't impose unacceptable burdens on others. The primary concern is that adults adequately protect their children's interests. If their claim is plausible, we think the analogous claim, about adequate would-be parents' rights to procreate a child in order to raise her, warrants investigation.

7. For the suggestion that reasons can be undercut by their interaction with moral considerations, see (McDowell, 1979; Raz, 1975, pp. 35–48). For the remainder of this article, we won't distinguish between the claim that the reasons in question are undercut (deprived of all normative force), and the claim that they are significantly attenuated (retaining some force but deprived of most of their strength). Readers unsympathetic to the undercutting and attenuation of reasons can recast our arguments as claims about the reason to procreate being outweighed by a stronger countervailing reason, without the reason to procreate being deprived of its normative force. On this revision of our view, we would deny that the parental relationship justification succeeds because the interests it highlights come into conflict with weighty moral considerations limiting how one can permissibly benefit from subjecting others to bad states.
8. There are strong reasons against government interference in people's sexual and procreative lives. However, this doesn't establish that there's a moral right to procreate, only that government should stay out of at least some aspects of the procreative realm.
9. At any rate, it could do so up to a certain point. Like Brighouse and Swift (2014, p. 56), we're concerned with defeasible rights, which can be overridden when there are sufficiently strong countervailing reasons (as when other rights are at stake).
10. On procreative ethics and environmental costs, see: MacIver (2015) and Young (2001).
11. Moreover, even if there is no moral right to procreate, many instances of procreation might still be permissible. Adults don't have a moral right to operate large trucks. As a result, it can be morally impermissible for them to do so if their operation will impose costs on others (e.g. risk of injury or property damage) that aren't paired with significant benefits. But it can also be perfectly permissible for some people to operate trucks when doing so isn't too costly for others and when the associated benefits are significant (as when trained drivers transport valuable items). The view we argue for here is that a particular justification of the moral right to procreate fails; even if there's no alternate argument for the right to procreate, this doesn't mean that procreation would always be impermissible, only that agents' procreation wouldn't be protected by a moral right.
12. Gheaus (in press) cites Brighouse and Swift's account of parental interests and the right to parent, and argues that it entails a right to procreate for adequate parents, when procreation is the necessary or best means to acquire a child to raise. Overall (2012) and Weinberg (2016) both argue that parental interests similar to those discussed by Brighouse and Swift provide the strongest reason for procreating. In an unpublished manuscript, Ferracioli (in press) articulates a parental interest justification that differs significantly from Brighouse and Swift's account of parental interests. Her account may avoid our challenge as a result (though we believe it has other problems that we can't take up here).
13. Children vary quite dramatically in their capacities, owing to genetic differences, environmental factors, and which developmental stage of childhood they occupy. Despite these differences, developmentally typical children of all ages are constituted so as to allow these special features of the parent–child relationship to manifest to some degree. This paper follows Brighouse and Swift in defining

children as 'people, who, because of their age, have yet to develop the capacities that characterize normal adulthood' (2014, p. 58).

14. We avoid discussion of how well-being should be understood in this paper, since we think the bads of childhood we discuss will be regarded as bad by many theories of well-being. While some views may not accept all of our explanations of why the states under consideration here are bad for children, we expect they will still accept enough of our claims to agree that (most of) the states are seriously bad for children to inhabit. That is enough for our purposes.
15. It is also, arguably, a form of domination, a fact which might compound the badness of parents' control of children. For a discussion of the claim that children are subject to the arbitrary will of parents, see Tomlin (in press).
16. 'An adult with supervisory power over a child has the power of life or death; and this is not, at least when the child is young, reciprocated. Less spectacularly, they have the power to make the child's life miserable or enjoyable (with limits, at least at the enjoyable end)' (Brighouse & Swift, 2014, p. 89).
17. For further discussion see Schapiro (1999).
18. There are concerns about whether this mode of thinking is coherent. For discussion, and a defense of the claim that creation can benefit, see Parfit (1984, pp. 487–490).

Acknowledgements

The authors share equal responsibility for this paper. We thank the following people for helpful comments on the ideas discussed here: Jaime Ahlberg, Clare Brennan, Mark Budolfson, Michael Cholbi, Ryan Cox, Russell DiSilvestro, Crystallene Fernando, Luara Ferracioli, Anca Gheaus, Dan Halliday, David Hills, Rob Kirby, Avery Kolers, Seth Lazar, Corey MacIver, Ben Miller, Rob Shaver, Liam Shields, Christine Sypnowich, Patrick Tomlin, and Richard Vernon. Thanks to Andrée-Anne Cormier and an anonymous reviewer at CRISPP for helpful referee reports. An anonymous reviewer elsewhere gave helpful comments on an earlier version. We also acknowledge audiences at: Australian National University, the Centre For Applied Philosophy and Public Ethics at Charles Stuart University, the 'From Procreative Acts to Parental Rights Workshop' at the University of Florida, University of Melbourne, University of Manitoba, the European Consortium for Political Research at the Université de Montréal, and the 'Permissible Progeny Workshop' and Rotman Institute of Philosophy at Western University. Sarah would like to thank the School of Philosophy at the Australian National University for hosting her as a visitor while she worked on this paper.

Disclosure statement

No potential conflict of interest was reported by the authors.

References

Brighouse, H., & Swift, A. (2014). *Family values: The ethics of parent-child relationships*. Princeton, NJ: Princeton University Press.

Ferracioli, L. (in press). Procreative-parenting, love's reasons and the demands of morality. *The Philosophical Quarterly*. doi:10.1093/pq/pqx022. Retrieved from https://academic.oup.com/pq/advance-article/doi/10.1093/pq/pqx022/3885959

Gheaus, A. (2011). Arguments for nonparental care for children. *Social Theory and Practice, 37*(3), 483–509.

Gheaus, A. (2015). The 'intrinsic goods of childhood' and the just society. In A. Bagattini & C. Macleod (Eds.), *The nature of children's well-being* (pp. 35–52). New York, NY: Springer.

Gheaus, A. (in press). The right to parent and duties concerning future generations. *Journal of Political Philosophy*. doi:10.1111/jopp.12091. Retrieved from http://onlinelibrary.wiley.com/doi/10.1111/jopp.12091/full

Hannan, S. (in press). Why Childhood is Bad for Children. *Journal of Applied Philosophy*. doi: 10.1111/japp.12256. Retrieved from http://onlinelibrary.wiley.com/wol1/doi/10.1111/japp.12256/full

MacIver, C. (2015). Procreation or appropriation? In S. Hannan, S. Brennan, & R. Vernon (Eds.), *Permissible progeny?: The morality of procreation and parenting* (pp. 107–128). New York, NY: Oxford University Press.

Macleod, C. (2010). Parental responsibilities in an unjust world. In D. Archard & D. Benatar (Eds.), *Procreation and parenthood: The ethics of bearing and rearing children* (pp. 128–150). Oxford: Oxford University Press.

Macleod, C. (2015). Agency, authority, and the vulnerability of children. In A. Bagattini & C. Macleod (Eds.), *The nature of children's well-being* (pp. 53–64). New York, NY: Springer.

McDowell, J. (1979). Virtue and reason. *The Monist, 62*(3), 35–48.

Overall, C. (2012). *Why have children?: The ethical debate*. Cambridge: MIT Press.

Parfit, D. (1984). *Reasons and persons*. Oxford: Oxford University Press.

Raz, J. (1975). *Practical reason and norms*. Oxford: Oxford University Press.

Schapiro, T. (1999). What is a child? *Ethics, 109*(4), 715–738.

Tomlin, P. (in press). Saplings or caterpillars?: Trying to understand children's wellbeing. *Journal of Applied Philosophy*. doi:10.1111/japp.12204. Retrieved from http://onlinelibrary.wiley.com/wol1/doi/10.1111/japp.12204/abstract

Weinberg, R. (2016). *The risk of a lifetime: How, when, and why procreation can be morally permissible*. Oxford: Oxford University Press.

Young, T. (2001). Overconsumption and procreation: Are they morally equivalent? *Journal of Applied Philosophy, 18*(2), 183–192.

Family values reconsidered: a response

Harry Brighouse and Adam Swift

ABSTRACT

It is wonderful to receive so much careful attention. But it's also frustrating. Each paper poses important questions, and between them they cover a wide range of issues. It is challenging, on such big topics, and in so few words, simultaneously to set the record straight, to identify the various objections posed by our critics, and to respond to them in a way likely to advance our collective understanding of the issues. Still, here goes.

The family and equality

In our book we, like a number of other theorists, frame the relationship between the family and justice in terms of a principle of equal opportunity. Rawls's interpretation of fair equal opportunity requires that people with similar native talents and willingness to use them should face roughly equal prospects for attaining valuable positions and the powers and prerogatives attached to them:

> The consistent application of the principle of fair opportunity requires us to view persons independently from the influences of their social position. But how far should this tendency be carried? It seems that even when fair opportunity (as it has been defined) is satisfied, the family will lead to unequal chances between individuals. Is the family to be abolished then?

His answer is that 'taken by itself and given a certain primacy, the idea of equal opportunity inclines in this direction' (1971, p. 511). Only the invocation of his other principles prevents this counter-intuitive result.

Anca Gheaus's paper (in press) is devoted to showing that even abolishing the family would not produce fair equality of opportunity. Colin Macleod (in press), by contrast, argues that the conflict between fair equality of opportunity and the family is less serious than we acknowledge. Both deny that fair equality of opportunity supports abolition, though in rather different ways. For Gheaus, it's because there will be unfair inequality of opportunity even with abolition, for Macleod it's because fair equality of opportunity can be achieved without it. We agree with Gheaus that alternative childrearing arrangements, and other forms of partiality, would continue to produce unfair inequalities of opportunity but we suspect that the latter would be considerably reduced. Macleod is right that in principle it is possible to reconcile the two, but we doubt that a just society would eliminate the conflict entirely.

It is important to see that fair equality of opportunity plays a strategic role in the exposition of our view: we employ it as the conventional example of the kind of impartial distributive principle with which familial partiality conflicts. We might have chosen other principles instead, perhaps a thoroughgoing luck egalitarianism, or a variant of prioritarianism such as the difference principle, or even a form of sufficientarianism. All of these can make demands on parents that seem to compete with their permissions, or even their obligations, to favor their children rather than others. Our aim was to identify the kinds of partiality that can be justified specifically by appeal to the value of the parent–child relationship, and our analysis would have been the same in all these cases.

Fair equality of opportunity seemed to us the strategic choice partly because of the way the Rawlsian frame has tended to structure academic discussion and partly because of that principle's wider intuitive appeal. Our aim was to identify a set of 'relationship goods,' and kinds of parent–child interaction productive of those goods, that should not be sacrificed to it despite that appeal, while arguing that the principle was important enough plausibly to constrain parents' attempts to confer advantage on their children in general. These expository benefits, for us, outweighed the principle's many defects, such as its limited specifications both of those whose opportunities should be equal and what those opportunities should be opportunities for, or the fact that our actual circumstances confront us with more urgent, impartially justified, distributive demands than those required by the principle (Brighouse & Swift, 2014, pp. 38–44, 143–145).

We argue that even if abolishing the family would result in fair equality of opportunity, abolition would not be justified, because the family provides important goods that are, from the impartial perspective, more important than fair equality of opportunity. So, if abolishing the family would not – even if it could not – make equality of opportunity possible, that does not affect our argument. According to Gheaus (in press), our analysis 'seems to rely on the assumption that, absent the family and other things being equal, there would be significantly less disruption of distributive justice.' If so, appearances are deceptive.

We make no empirical assumption of that kind. More, we do not suppose that familial partiality is the only kind of partiality that is *legitimate*, nor even that it is the kind of legitimate partiality that is, empirically, most likely to disrupt fair equality of opportunity. Our aim is to show that parent–child relationships justify less conferral of advantage than is commonly thought, and provide less by way of justified opposition to egalitarian policies than is commonly acknowledged. It is compatible with this that *other* relationships might justify extensive partiality of a kind that interfered with fair equality of opportunity, and that justified resistance to egalitarian policies. To investigate whether other forms of relationship, such as friendship or compatriotism or co-religiosity, would justify such interference and resistance one would need, on our approach, to consider the specificity of those relationships and think about what kinds of partiality might be defended by appeal to the goods they produce.[1] It is true that we, like many others, regard the familial case as generating particularly important permissions and requirements, and we are doubtful that careful examination of the goods produced by these other relationships will show their production to legitimate extensive expressions of partiality of the kind that would disrupt fair equality of opportunity – or other impartial principles. But our book does not take a stand on that, separate, question.[2]

Nothing in our view denies that, in the absence of the family, people would act in ways just as disruptive of fair equality of opportunity as they do in its presence. Perhaps, deprived of their ability to confer advantage on their children, people might be even more keenly motivated to benefit their friends, their compatriots or their co-religionists. Similarly, for our (limited, specific) purposes, one does not need to know if 'alternative childrearing institutions would be significantly less likely to disrupt fair distributions than a (properly reformed) family' (Gheaus, in press, p. xx).

When thinking about this empirical counterfactual, one must keep clear that a 'properly reformed' family would already be likely to be less disruptive (though not, perhaps, less likely to be disruptive) of that principle than the family as it exists at moment. (If, as Macleod and we suggest, the wider society were also subject to egalitarian reform, that would do even more to reduce the conflict.) We certainly agree with Gheaus that any system of childrearing that might plausibly serve the relevant interests at all well could not, for the reasons she gives, be expected to give all children equality of opportunity for jobs and the rewards that attach to them. There would of course be innumerable contingencies at the individual level – some adults will just be a better fit with some children – but how much inequality of opportunity could be *expected* will depend on a number of variables, particularly, perhaps, the extent of variation in the relevant adults' child rearing capacities (which we assume would be less than between parents in even the properly reformed family), and the number of children each adult would raise over her lifetime (which we assume would be more).[3] Given less variation in parenting input and less exclusive attention to particular children, we hazard that a system of the kind she has in mind would tend to produce less inequality of opportunity than even a properly reformed family. It is an interesting, and different, question what kinds of partiality could be *justified* by appeal to the adult–child relationships in question. The first step in thinking about that would be to clarify the nature of those relationships, especially how exactly they differ from the parent–child relationship in the properly reformed family.[4]

Macleod is surely right that there is no necessary conflict between the family and fair equality of opportunity. One way to see this is simply to imagine a society in which children are raised in families but there is no overall inequality in the rewards, both intrinsic (e.g. self-realization) and extrinsic (e.g. income), that attach to different jobs; there would still be different jobs and children would doubtless have unequal chances of achieving them, but there would be no inequality of prospects with respect to rewards. Or suppose that jobs were unequally rewarded but people were allocated to them randomly, or by other mechanisms that rendered irrelevant the way they had been raised as children. These possibilities suffice to establish his claim, though he has in mind a different reconciliatory, less outlandish, scenario: a 'non-hierarchical community' in which parents are more equal with respect to childrearing ability and motivation, public institutions help to mitigate any residual inequalities in children's competences, and a wide range of different skills are valued by society.

Macleod very nicely brings out the contingency of the empirical differences and inequalities that in fact generate the conflict between the family and fair equality of opportunity. Where we emphasized that contingency especially with respect to children's outcomes (Brighouse & Swift, 2014, pp. 129–130), he mainly focuses on parental – and other – inputs. Still, we doubt that the family and fair equality of opportunity could be entirely reconciled in a *just* society, because we think that justice requires the permission of at least somewhat unequal inputs and outcomes. Indeed, fair equality of opportunity itself is plausibly construed as requiring that permission.[5] Although strictly speaking that principle is entirely negative, objecting solely to people's prospects being affected by their social class background, it is normally understood also as permitting, and on some interpretations even requiring, that those prospects indeed be influenced by their natural talents and willingness to use them. In any case, any plausible specification of the principle will leave individuals, however equal their prospects, free to make choices – about what kind of work to do, for example, or how hard to work, or how to spend their leisure time (Brighouse & Swift, 2014, p. 30). At least some of those choices will properly leave them unequal, or at least different, with respect to attributes that may legitimately affect their interactions with their children in ways that it is in practice impossible to prevent from impacting somewhat on those children's prospects, if their children's own freedom to make choices, when capable of so doing, is also to be respected.

We might put it this way. Nothing about *family values* prevents the achievement of fair equality of opportunity. There is, on our view, no parental right to confer advantage, or to have parent–child interactions that are properly protected (such as bedtime stories) rewarded in a way that conflicts with that principle. It is other, more general, considerations that generate the conflict. Like Macleod, we think that, compared both to conventional views and to the status quo in most affluent societies, the conflict between the family and fair equality of opportunity can be significantly mitigated – as indeed can the conflict between the family and other impartial distributive principles. Unlike him, we doubt that a just society could eliminate it altogether.

Parenting and perfectionism

Our book tries to tread a careful line on one of the most fundamental issues in political philosophy: whether it is proper for the state to act on judgments about the content of a good life, or whether it should aim rather to provide a just framework that remains neutral between them.[6] Our theory as a whole certainly has mildly perfectionist elements but, as Christine Sypnowich (in press) observes, we are at pains to emphasize how much of the argument does not depend on them. From her avowedly perfectionist perspective, this looks like backsliding, and a missed opportunity: our argument 'makes it clear that political philosophy has been impoverished for its jettisoning of questions of human flourishing' (p. xx); the faces exuding wellbeing in the Norman Rockwell painting on the cover need no anti-perfectionist caveats.[7]

In this section we explain our reluctance to be cast as flag bearers for perfectionism, and try to clarify where perfectionist elements do indeed play a role in the argument. While we are readier to disown those elements than she would like, she is quicker to see them than we think warranted. The justification of policies aimed at promoting or supporting family life is a very important topic, so it matters to have a clear picture of the structure of the issues. By setting out our version of that picture, we hope at least to enable those who disagree with us to understand where, and why, they do so.

We downplay the importance of the perfectionist strands in the argument for two reasons (Brighouse & Swift, 2014, pp. 178–181). On the one hand, we don't want convinced anti-perfectionists to dismiss our views on the mistaken assumption that they are irredeemably and entirely perfectionist. Generally, whatever one's conclusions, one wants arguments that are austere, appealing to premises that are no more controversial than necessary. In so far as we can articulate a theory of the value of the family, and of its implications for policy, without appealing to judgments that some will reject outright and others will regard as inappropriate bases for political action, we would want to do that. It is a very good question exactly how much of our theory does indeed survive, as a contribution to political theory, without those bases, and one that we hope the following discussion will better enable us, and others, to answer.

On the other hand, we feel the force of neutralist considerations. Sypnowich thinks that our sympathetic characterization of anti-perfectionism 'caricatures' (p. xx) perfectionist views, but we stand by it (2014, p. 178). Even a mild, pluralistic perfectionism like ours does indeed use the coercive power of the state, if only through tax and subsidy, on behalf of some ways of living rather than others, and there are various difficult questions – e.g. about the state's capacity to make those judgments well, or about what constitutes equal respect for citizens – that make us less ready than her simply to assume the propriety of perfectionist state action. The case for neutralism is, we believe, powerful enough for us to want to show how much of our argument would continue to apply if it were valid.

Sypnowich thinks that we invoke perfectionist arguments in our case for the value of familial relationships for both children and parents (in press). While the weighty and non-substitutable interest in parenting that we identify does indeed claim to specify an element in a flourishing life for many adults, we are not convinced that the account of children's interests to which we appeal violates an anti-perfectionist constraint. And even if our full account of why children need parents does violate it, it remains important to see that even neutralists can accept child-centered arguments for the family – and for the 'relationship goods' it produces.

We appeal to five interests of children to justify the family (and ground the child's right to a parent): four of these relate to various aspects of children's development (physical, cognitive, emotional, and moral), the fifth concerns the quality of their childhood as such (Brighouse & Swift, 2014, p. 64).[8] We shall not repeat here how the argument goes, though we will stress that the interrelationships between the interests are crucial. For current purposes, what's important is that three of these interests satisfy anti-perfectionist criteria in a very straightforward way: even neutralists can and do think it a proper task for the state to help future citizens develop their physical, cognitive and moral capacities. Emotional development is perhaps a little more controversial, but we deliberately specify it very broadly and, importantly, give no special place to the development of the capacity for distinctively *familial* relationships.[9] Perhaps some variants of anti-perfectionism would regard even this as beyond the pale, but we suspect that more plausible versions will either accept it as appropriately neutral between conceptions of wellbeing or see it as presupposed by the kind of interest (e.g. in framing, revising and pursuing a conception of the good, or in acting on one's sense of justice) that neutralists can endorse. Childhood goods are an interesting case. In so far as they are valuable on these other developmental grounds, they too are presupposed. Where they are intrinsically valuable, the fact that anti-perfectionists are primarily concerned with people's attributes as adults leaves their status unclear to us. Perhaps it is impossible to have an anti-perfectionist understanding of a good childhood – any such understanding will rest on a fuller theory of human flourishing than the neutralist can accept. Or perhaps common sense understandings of such a childhood do not violate anti-perfectionist strictures.

Whatever one thinks about this last issue, we believe that familial relationships of the kind we describe are justified even by appeal to what we might call children's 'neutral interests.' At times Sypnowich seems to conflate paternalism and perfectionism, detecting exceptions to neutralism where none exist; even the resolute anti-perfectionist can recognize that children differ from adults in ways that justify the paternalistic treatment of the former but not the latter (p. xx). Similarly, one should not read all talk of providing children with an upbringing that is conducive to their flourishing as betraying perfectionist leanings. On our understanding, the anti-perfectionist can hold that the state – and perhaps even parents – are properly guided by a concern that children live flourishing lives, and can act paternalistically towards that end, provided that that concern does not take a determinate view about what counts as flourishing. The capacity for autonomy, for example, can be an appropriate guide to political action, even to the neutralist, partly because of its connection to flourishing, if those who have it are best placed to judge wherein their own flourishing consists.

Where children's interest in being parented can, we believe, generate the case for familial relationships of the kind that we describe without violating anti-perfectionist constraints, our articulation of adults' interest in being parents does take us into avowedly perfectionist territory – at least when we argue that it can properly guide state policy. Where the rights *of* parents (a.k.a. 'parents' rights') are justified entirely by appeal to children's interests, which could be construed in neutralist terms, the right *to* parent depends on a claim about the weighty and non-substitutable contribution to adults' wellbeing made by a rather particular kind of relationship: one in which the adult acts as the child's fiduciary and successfully discharges her fiduciary duties by having an intimate-but-authoritative loving relationship with the child.[10] When we argue that society should support adults in their attempts to become parents, indeed when we argue that those adults who are good enough parents have an interest that defeats a child's claim to the best available parent, we are invoking a perfectionist claim about the value of parenting. *That* claim, indeed, is unusually fully specified. Not only do we, unlike (e.g.) Nussbaum, regard parenting as *sui generis* – rather than subsumable into the general category of emotional life – which might already be enough to violate some neutralist constraints; we also offer a very specific articulation of the value of parenting, and one that others have seen much to quarrel with (see, for example, Ferracioli, 2016, in press; Reshef, 2013).

As in our previous remarks, it is important, however, to see that the case for regarding familial relationship goods as distribuenda, and for advocating policies – flexible working arrangements, home visits, even workshops on reading bedtime stories (p. xx) – aiming at their more equal distribution does not depend entirely on adults' interest in parenting, or in parenting well. Certainly, we believe that those interests may legitimately be taken into account by policymakers, but we would be disappointed if readers came away with the impression that they play a crucial role in that strand of our argument. Policies of that kind can often be justified by appeal to children's 'neutral' interests. To parent is to play a fiduciary role for one's children; to parent well is to do that well. The case for more equal distributions of familial relationship goods, or indeed for distributions meeting sufficientarian desiderata, depends primarily on the claims of *children*. We could, to be sure, formulate the case in terms of the distribution of opportunities for flourishing, as Sypnowich urges us to, but we have suggested that doing so need involve no perfectionist commitments. Claims in favor of state support for artificial reproductive technology, or of giving adults' interests any weight in the design of adoption policies, are different. Those do appeal to a specific view about adult wellbeing of the kind that she would like to see more of.

Sharing and shaping values

In *Family Values* we tackle the question of the extent to which parents may legitimately share their values with, and shape the values of, their children. This is obviously an area where the will of parents and the interests of children are potentially in conflict. We argue that, for several familiar reasons, children have an interest in becoming autonomous adults – equipped with the intellectual and emotional resources to make and, over time, rationally to revise, considered and careful judgments about what values should guide their lives, and about what to do in particular circumstances. Society has an interest in children being constrained not only by the law but by internalized dispositions to treat others justly, honestly and with respect. But parents normally seek, and may well have an interest in, sharing their lives with their children, in ways that inevitably end up shaping those children's values. Shaping values while fostering autonomy is not necessarily impossible, but it certainly creates a potential for tension.

Daniel Weinstock (in press) observes that the subtitle of our book is *The Ethics of Parent–Child Relationships* and argues that we also need a *political philosophy* of parent–child relationships. Social institutions that supplement the family can address the tensions between the parental will to shape values and the child's interest in autonomy; schools in particular should play a major role in fostering autonomy. Andrée-Anne Cormier's paper (in press) also concerns this conflict. Whereas Sypnowich urges us to be more, or more openly, perfectionist, Cormier pursues a version of the argumentative strategy suggested above: parents' deliberately shaping their children's values in the light of their comprehensive views can sometimes be justified by appeal to children's 'neutral' interest in developing autonomy, so does not violate any anti-perfectionist constraint.

We find Cormier's paper elegant and congenial. Much of it is a critique of Matthew Clayton's view on these issues, and we look forward to his response. But reflecting on her anti-perfectionist defense of our position has led us to identify some lack of clarity in one aspect of the view as presented in our book.[11] In *Family Values* we argue that parents have an obligation to shape some of their children's values – those that will enable and incline them to treat others justly, and to behave well as citizens. This obligation, and the content of the values, is entirely independent of the values that parents distinctively hold. But parents also have a limited right to shape their children's values in ways that reflect their own. The right is limited primarily by a concern for the child's interest in developing autonomy, the facilitation of which is also a parental obligation. That right is our focus here. The argument we present grounds the right in familial relationship goods and appeals primarily to the importance, for children, of parents' being free to be spontaneously intimate and to share themselves with their child: part of feeling free to be spontaneous is not engaging in the excessive self-monitoring that would be required to shield the child from all one's interests and values. But we also defend some deliberate shaping of children's values, where that is necessary for the development and maintenance – including maintenance into adulthood – of an intimate familial relationship. Such a relationship requires at least some shared distinctive values, which in the early part of childhood, at least, will typically come from the adult.

Cormier argues that this second, deliberate, class of value-shaping can be defended on anti-perfectionist grounds where it is necessary for the kind of familial relationship that is itself conducive to children's developmental interests, most notably their interest in developing autonomy. She thinks that children would retrospectively consent to having their values deliberately shaped where that is the case. Indeed, she canvasses the further possibility that parents' enrolling children into their own comprehensive doctrines may itself be defended in this way.

To clarify the issues raised by her paper, note that there are key differences, some of which are obscured rather than clarified by our discussion in the book (Brighouse & Swift, 2014, pp. 154–157), between (i) parents' *spontaneously* sharing/revealing their values, (ii) parents' *deliberately* sharing/revealing their values, and (iii) parents' deliberately *aiming to influence* their children's values. Taking one's child to church can be a deliberate way of introducing them to a belief system and a set of practices that one judges valuable and wants to share with one's children but, in principle at least, it need not involve any attempt deliberately to influence the values they come to hold; it need not be a deliberate attempt to get them to endorse Christianity. It is, to be sure, deliberate rather than spontaneous. But the aim is, or can be, merely that of revealing who one is to – sharing one's enthusiasms with – one's children. There need be no intention to guarantee, or even to increase the likelihood of, their coming to endorse those values.

Of course, *all* these classes of parent–child interaction will have the *effect* of shaping children's values. And even in class (ii), the parent might presumably *hope* that the child will come to endorse the values that the parent is revealing to her. Indeed, as Weinstock emphasizes, one may worry about the autonomy-inhibiting impact of all three classes, with serious repercussions for the parental duty of care to facilitate children's autonomy. But, bracketing that concern, the difficult question raised by Cormier's argument concerns which of them can be really be justified by appeal to familial relationship goods and the developmental interests that they serve.

How should we think about cases of the kind she describes here?:

> For some parents – perhaps especially religiously committed parents – comprehensively enrolling their children, e.g. by baptizing them, bringing them to church and teaching them the value of things like spirituality, or family ties, or love, as they understand it in light of their religious view, may not only be an important source of fulfillment and joy, but also a key and indispensible element of what it means for them to be authentic in building a connection with their children. (p. xx)

One might consider a parent who can only connect authentically with her child by engaging in these kinds of interaction to have misunderstood the duties of parenthood. That would be analogous to our view that a parent who cuts off relations with a child who rejects the parent's religion has misunderstood her role (Brighouse & Swift, 2014, p. 157). In such cases, familial relationship goods are at the mercy of whatever parents need to connect authentically with their children, which may be true empirically but is problematic as a justification of the interaction. We can indeed imagine a child saying to her parent:

> I understand why you brought me up to believe in the Bible. Given your beliefs, that was the only way for us to have the kind of close loving relationship I needed to have with you if I was going to develop the autonomy I am now able to exercise (and which I exercise by rejecting Christianity).

But it is hard not to think that there is something wrong with the parents' beliefs in that case. Just as, on our view, parents can enjoy loving familial relationships with their children without acting on their entirely natural desire generally to confer (unjustly advantageous) benefits on them, so, perhaps, they can enjoy such relationships without acting on their desire, perhaps also entirely natural, to try to get their children to endorse the same values as them. A fuller exploration of these issues would – we hope will – take another paper, exploring, in addition to the distinctions set out above, the differences between (a) revealing one's values, (b) getting one's children to participate in practices implied by those values, and (c) attempting to influence the values that one's children endorse, whether during their childhoods or as the adults they will become.

In the book we frequently deploy a distinction between what people should be permitted to do *qua* parents, *on family values grounds*, and what they should be permitted to do *all things considered*. To the frustration of those quite reasonably interested in the latter issue, our focus is the former; we are concerned specifically with those parent–child interactions that are 'susceptible to justification by appeal to the parent–child relationship' (Brighouse & Swift, 2014, p. 146).[12] So it is not altogether surprising that our theory supports only a right to do those things that are necessary in order for the relationship to flourish. Still, the amount of sharing that is necessary might be considerable. And it is worth remembering that a good deal of deliberate value-shaping – that required to ensure that the children will grow up with a sense of justice – is obligatory. Success in *that* value-shaping task probably takes a good deal of intimacy and connectedness between parents and children, especially in social contexts where justice values are not well supported by the broader, extra-familial, environment: the showing of examples, modeling of behavior, and exposure to other models of behavior, might be more effective in the context of shared 'discretionary' valuing. And, as long as it is consistent with the development of the child's autonomy, more sharing, and perhaps even intentional shaping, might be legitimate on other grounds that we do not consider.

Weinstock notes that our commitment to the prospective autonomy of the child limits the ways in which parents may deliberately shape their children's values, and even the spontaneity with which they may share them. He takes us to hold that parents should not 'exert emotional pressure' on their children, pointing out that:

> a parent who in the presence of her children displays enthusiasm and passion in engaging in the activities that she finds valuable is, by this very fact, exerting emotional pressure upon her children. If her relationship with her children is healthy, then they will tend to be emotionally disposed to find pleasing the things their parents take pleasure in. When parents act on this disposition, whether they do so intentionally or not, they are exercising emotional pressure. And yet they are doing something that would seem to be called for by the theory of familial intimacy under discussion. (p. xx)

We agree, and say so (Brighouse & Swift, 2014, pp. 172–173). Our claim about emotional pressure is specifically that the complex and burdensome duty that parents are under with respect to value sharing and value-shaping includes 'restraining themselves from exerting the emotional pressure that they may be tempted deliberately to impose on the child to refrain from revising her received commitments' (p. 173). Some degree of pressure is indeed surely unavoidable. When it comes to a love of cricket, or an enthusiasm for hip-hop music, it is not at all hard to imagine a parent who sincerely and in good faith will not have the slightest disappointment if her child fails to come to share that love or enthusiasm. But that attitude is more difficult to adopt in the case of religious or political values and commitments. And even in the former case, even emotionally well-balanced children may well anticipate, contrary to fact, that rejection of the enthusiasm will provoke disappointment.

Weinstock (in press) claims that 'this juggling act between intimacy and autonomy' is not required of families:

> We need not look to just one institution, such as the family, as the sine qua non of the child's autonomy. We need not impose upon it the responsibility of ensuring that the children that are raised within it are raised autonomously. Nor do we need to overtax the state's capacity by requiring that in the name of the autonomy of children it observe the ways in which they are raised by parents in the intimate sphere. Nor need the state stand ready to intervene in that sphere when children are subject to value-shaping which, though it cannot be qualified as brainwashing or rank manipulation, may perhaps be viewed as excessive from the point of view of a parenting ethics that requires of parents that they attend both to ensuring that familial relations are characterized by the requisite degree of intimacy, and that it be a locus for the teaching of autonomous-decision-making.

The solution, for him, lies in state-regulated, autonomy-promoting schools. These need not teach the value of autonomy directly; it is enough that they meet the negative condition of 'not simply being extensions of the values around which the familial domain is organized' (p. xx).

Again, we agree with much of this; we never suggest that it is parents' responsibility, on their own, to ensure their children's autonomy. Indeed, one of us (Brighouse, 1998, 2005, 2006) has argued extensively that schools play a valuable, maybe essential, role in facilitating children's autonomy, even for families that are entirely committed to their children's autonomy, and that a key feature of an autonomy-facilitating school will be an ethos which is somewhat 'discontinuous' from that of the home and the mainstream culture. It is through schooling that the state is most easily able to supply the raw materials needed for autonomy: through the curriculum and high quality instruction children can experience intellectual and emotional encounters with ideas, values, and traditions that are different from, and sometimes conflict with, those they are raised with in the home. Perhaps more importantly, in a socially and culturally diverse school they can become acquainted with different ideas, values and traditions through the friendships they make and through intimate interactions with their friends' families. A culturally diverse teaching force can provide children with a range of adult role models who are unlike them and whom they can come to admire. A robust and well-designed extra-curriculum can lead them to discover enthusiasms and interests that would never have been stimulated by their home culture.

Still, we sound a couple of notes of caution. The first is simply that one should not overestimate the state's capacity to provide the kind of schooling that will facilitate autonomy, even for children whose parents are not hostile to it, let alone for those whose parents resist their development as independent persons. In any society that values autonomy, consumer choice is likely to play a considerable role in the allocation of various goods, including housing and schooling, and markets are liable to play a large role in the allocation of jobs. This can make it very difficult to achieve a mix of cultures within schools, either among the staff or among the students, especially (but not only) in areas with lower population density. Even when cultural diversity among the student population is achieved, children's tendency to prefer to socialize with others who pretty much like them makes it difficult to harness that diversity as an aid to autonomy, which may often reasonably be a lesser priority than improving students' academic outcomes. Teachers tend to mirror the general population in terms of their political, religious, and cultural outlooks, so it is not surprising that in many schools the ethos is not at all discontinuous with the culture of that of most of the homes of the students who attend. Equipping teachers with the skills necessary for teaching basic mathematics, science, and reading is already a difficult task. Equipping them to enable children to reflect critically and well not only on the values they have been raised with but also on the, possibly autonomy-eroding, values that permeate the mainstream ethos of modern capitalist societies – which many of those teachers unreflectively endorse – is more challenging still.

The second note of caution is that, however useful a political philosophy of parent–child relationships might be, an ethics of parent–child relationships remains essential. Even high quality schooling for autonomy would not eliminate the 'juggling act between intimacy and autonomy' that Weinstock seems to think that we can avoid requiring of families. Parents who are determined to resist autonomy can adopt strategies to immunize their children from the autonomy-promoting lessons and experiences that the school provides. Those strategies may sometimes fail, but they will succeed often enough for parents' choices about how to respond to schools' attempts to promote critical reflection on the values they themselves hold to remain important. Even where parents make no deliberate attempts at immunization, the emotional pull of their parents' enthusiasms will be enough to prevent many children from responding to the schools' messages. This is especially likely if parents take the awareness that another institution is taking care of autonomy as entitling them to be completely uninhibited in their promotion of their own values. And because, as Weinstock acknowledges, it is important that schools not damage healthy familial relationships, the autonomy-promoting role of schools itself places limits on what parents may teach children at home. So consider the parents who, thinking themselves freed from the responsibility for promoting their child's autonomy by the presence of an autonomy-facilitating school, teach her that homosexuality, or apostasy, are sins punishable by eternal damnation. One can easily imagine that what the school would have to do to facilitate that child's autonomy would interfere with the familial relationship. We see no way that parents can be relieved of the duty to participate conscientiously in developing their child's autonomy.

If that is right, then we have to accept that parents have obligations that the state cannot enforce. We agree with Weinstock (in press, p. xx) that 'the line distinguishing acceptable from unacceptable kinds of value-forming would simply escape states' epistemic capacity, even for states that had eschewed liberal democratic concerns with excessive surveillance of its citizenry.' For us, the importance of intimacy within the parent–child relationships means that parents must be given space within which they can, in fact, fail to deliver on their duties. We do not see a way around this.

Procreation and childhood

We hardly discuss procreation in *Family Values*. We argue that adults have an interest in *parenting*, explain what that interest consists in, and claim that it is weighty enough to support a prima facie right to parent. We assume a continuing supply of children needing parents, and that childhood is a natural biological condition with the properties that enable adults to realize the interest in parenting, and through which all human beings lucky enough to reach adulthood will pass. But we do not even argue that procreation is ever justified, all things considered. If, for example, we agreed with David Benatar (2008) that most lives are not worth living, because they contain more bad than good for the people living them, we would think that was a strong reason for most people not to procreate, despite the interest in parenting. We do not agree with him about that. More particularly, because we do not claim that the adult interest in parenting includes the interest in parenting a genetic descendent, we do not argue that adults are justified in procreating in order to fulfill their own interest in parenting.

Sarah Hannan and R.J. Leland (in press) are therefore not criticizing us directly when they challenge the view that the interest in parenting is strong enough to establish a right to procreate. But their argument is implicitly critical of us for the tacit assumptions we make about childhood: that it is a stage of life, that is usually, or at least often, well worth experiencing and going through. This gives us an opportunity to discuss further the nature of childhood, and its relationship to the interest in parenting.

Hannan and Leland observe that for adults to fulfill the interest we describe in parenting a child they need to be supplied with beings with certain features: viz., impaired practical reason, a need for extensive parental control, profound and asymmetric vulnerability, and no established practical identity. We agree. Hannan and Leland claim, though, that these are bad-making features of a life and, in particular, that possessing these features is bad for children. Because they are bad for children, the adult interest in relationships with beings that possess these features cannot form the basis of a justification for procreation, let alone of a right to procreate. But we think several responses are available to someone who, unlike us, wanted to use the adult interest to play that justificatory role.

The first would be to concede that the features of childhood to which they point are, indeed, bad, but observe that the parent's job is to deliver children from that condition. On this view it would be a matter of good fortune that the purportedly bad-making features of childhood make parenting distinctively rewarding, because this gives children a reasonably reliable way of escaping it. We give considerable emphasis to the interest parents have in raising children to become autonomous, independent adults, and the distinctive challenge posed by that particular task. For adults to enjoy the goods of parenting, those who are parented must have the capacity, if the role is discharged only reasonably well, to develop into adults whose practical reasoning is mature, who no longer need parental control and are no longer profoundly or asymmetrically vulnerable and who have a well-developed practical identity. An important part of what it is to realize the interest in parenting is to oversee the child's development to this adult state. Parenting, on our stipulation, is not a matter of caring for someone who lacks the capacity to develop into an adult: the role is to oversee that development.

As they figure in our account of the value of parenting, the purportedly bad-making features of childhood are, then, temporary, transient and necessary steps on the path to adulthood. So creating a child whom one knows will have these purportedly bad-making features with the reasonable expectation that they will be transcended through the process of parenting is quite different from producing a child that one knows will never develop into adulthood, and that one will control it for all of its life. To do *that* would indeed be to treat those features of childhood that make it bad for children as one's reason for procreation. But the interest in parenting is not simply an interest in exploiting the bad-for-children properties for one's own sake. It is an interest in being the person who has the kind of relationship with the child that serves his interest in becoming an adult.

A second, and related, response would insist that, for us, the adult interest in parenting is misunderstood if it is conceived primarily as an interest in having control over another being, or in having another being dependent on oneself. Its core is an interest in a particular kind of loving relationship: a unique combination of intimacy and fiduciary authority. It is *what* children need from parents if they are to develop into adults that make parenting distinctively and importantly valuable for adults. Children need

> a special kind of *relationship* – a relationship in which the adults offers love and authority, a complex and emotionally challenging combination of openness and restraint, of spontaneity and self-monitoring, of sharing and withholding. It's that kind of relationship that adults have an interest in too. (Brighouse & Swift, 2014, p. 93, original emphasis)

Anyone who parents, or procreates, simply so that she can exercise control over a dependent has got something very badly wrong.

But we want to respond a bit more forcefully by doubting that the features of childhood that make a parental relationship with a child valuable for adults are, in fact, bad for children. On the contrary, we suggest that these are good-making features, both for the child during her childhood and for the adult she will become.

It would be nice to frame our discussion of these features in terms of the 'childhood goods' or the 'special' or 'intrinsic' goods of childhood that they make possible (Brennan, 2014; Gheaus, 2015a, 2015b). We lack, alas, the control to do that well, partly because we are not yet clear on how that category is best understood. Are they those features and goods, possessed by or available to children but not adults, that are intrinsically valuable for children – i.e. good for children during their childhoods, irrespective of any instrumental or developmental benefits? The test for those would be to consider whether someone who died on the cusp of adulthood had benefitted from having the properties in question. Or are they those features and goods, possessed by or available to children, but not adults, that are valuable for people to have as children because they make possible the kind of development that is good for the adults they become? In practice, we suspect, many such properties and goods are both; for example, it is good for adults that they were unselfconsciously playful as children – it enabled the kind of development that benefitted them as adults – but unselfconscious playfulness is 'intrinsically' good for children too (i.e. it is good for them even if they are not lucky enough to live to become the adults who would have benefitted from being playful children).

That said, let's start with dependence on another person for having one's needs met and the necessity of parental control. After a long period of independence such a situation might indeed be undignified, or frustrating. But for a child, at the beginning of a full life, it enables her to enjoy experiences that would otherwise be unavailable or, perhaps, only insecurely available. Children can be – and many are, at least in reasonably favorable circumstances – carefree in a way that adults typically cannot. That experience – of going through a day without worrying about one's own future, one's responsibilities to others, the horrors one will encounter in the world beyond – is precious, and is facilitated by being in the state of vulnerability that makes one need loving, caring, and stable parental control. One of the reasons, furthermore, why that experience is so rare in adulthood is that our established practical identities involve us in a web of mutual responsibility; for the flourishing adult who relates successfully to others' carefreeness must be rare and fleeting, precisely because it is a holiday from her practical identity.

Like dependence, children's being 'primed' for spontaneous and unconditional trust and love enables them to enjoy experiences that are unavailable later in life, once one has got the measure of the world and all its possible disappointments. The child who, without self-consciousness and with complete spontaneity, dances when a parent returns from a short trip and then throws himself into a hug is experiencing something distinctively valuable that is only possible due to the character of his love.

Now think about the alleged defect of lacking an established practical identity. This feature of childhood is a precondition for the good of *developing an established practical identity*. As children and adolescents we undergo a large and complex variety of learning experiences, including the gradual discovery of what our interests are, of what we are truly like, of what other people are like and how to read them well, of intense bouts of friendship some of which, even if brief, have lifelong impacts on us, of discovery of features of the world that are fascinating, or dreary, or sublime. Throughout childhood we have innumerable learning experiences, some distressing, many challenging, and many more intensely rewarding (including many of those that are also distressing and challenging). These all contribute to the development of a practical identity and would be different, and in many cases less valuable, experiences if we already had one. In adulthood we (usually, more or less) know who we are and allow our interests and identities to filter out important features of the natural and social world. We wear blinkers because we are no longer embarked on a journey of discovery while mapping the world and finding our place in it; though revising our views of course remains possible, as adults what we are usually doing is more like finding and following directions to where we want to go. That experience – the mapping of the world – is impossible if we already have an established practical identity.

Try to think, now, about the alternative: entering the world *with* an established practical identity. In fact, as we'll suggest later, we're not sure we can make sense of this possibility for beings like us. But in so far as we can, the established practical identity would have to be given, either by some creator, or by nature. In either case, there is an important sense in which it would not be ours. Our practical identities become ours – and established as ours – through a process in which we experience and interact with countless environmental influences and other persons, some of which touch us profoundly, others of which barely touch us, and many of which fall somewhere in between. Exactly how each interaction influences us is affected by what else has happened, by what the other influences have been and will be, and by the character of our, particular, embodied, emerging practical identity. What enables us to be autonomous is that our practical identities are not given by a creator, by our parents, or by nature, but develop and are established through childhood and into adulthood, as well as being revised through our adult lives.[13]

Even impaired practical reason is valuable. Patrick Tomlin (2016) amusingly speculates that we might feel sorry for children because they are both so pleased, and so upset, by things that just do not matter. But while we would – and do – indeed feel sorry for adults afflicted with that tendency, we are inclined rather to envy children's capacity to be so affected by trivial things. To be so readily distressed might, taken on its own, be regrettable, even for a child, but to be so easily thrilled and joyful seems to us fortunate. To be sure, there might be children who are *so* quickly prone to excessive emotional reactions that they would be better off on a more even keel – if only because such a disposition is tiring and liable to get in the way of other valuable elements in their lives. But, assuming that the capacity for irrational suffering and joy come together as a package, we are generally inclined to envy children their capacity rather than feel sorry for them.

Somebody might object that we romanticize childhood – either here, or in our book. But we don't. Childhood is marked by features that are valuable at that stage in life, both because they make possible valuable experiences during childhood and because they are developmentally valuable; we have particularly emphasized the development that makes our established practical identities our own. But, of course, the valuable experiences and development these features facilitate depend on the cooperation of the world. Being dependent on adults for one's wellbeing is bad for you if no adult cares to, and is competent to, look after you. The seriously impaired rationality of a toddler can be *disastrous* in a world of unfenced precipices and inattentive adults.

A final comment. It is tempting to think about the issue of whether childhood is bad for children by asking whether it would be better for human beings to emerge into the world as fully formed adults. Hannan and Leland invite this question with their example of Dr. Frankensteen's creation, Monstra. Monstra could have been created as a fully formed adult, but Frankensteen chose instead to endow her with a nature such that she would go through a lengthy period of child-like dependence in order to provide him with a parent-like experience.

In so far as we can make sense of the question we don't think it would be better for human beings to emerge into the world as fully formed adults. But we resist the question. As our discussion above indicates, we are not sure what it would mean to be an agent, or to have an established practical identity, if one emerged into the world as an adult. Human beings – the kinds of beings for which all of the resources of moral theorizing that we know of have been developed – are organic. They emerge into the world helpless, and their development into adulthood involves physical, cognitive, and emotional growth in an appropriately nurturing and cooperative environment. They enter adulthood endowed with knowledge, skills, dispositions, attitudes, relationships, and memories that have developed over the course of their childhood through interactions with the world beyond their bodies. These attributes, including the relationships and memories, are not incidental to their selves, but partly constitutive of them. While we have played along with the thought that persons might be able to avoid childhood and its purportedly bad-making features for the sake of arguing that those features are not, in fact, bad, we are not sure that we can really make sense of it.

Conclusion

It's true that we have more to say. But we make no pretense that only considerations of space have prevented us from providing better responses to the six papers assembled in this special issue. We have been given much to ponder, and have been prompted to engage with difficult and complex issues, some of which had been more or less consciously sidestepped or pushed under the carpet, some of which had never occurred to us. Properly to engage with the full range of questions raised by our critics will take not only more words but also a good deal more work. We are extremely grateful to all the contributors, both for their careful attention and for pressing us to wade into deeper waters. We hope to come up with more satisfactory answers in due course.

Notes

1. Which is not to say that all partiality must be justified by appeal to relationship goods of any kind. See Brighouse and Swift (2015, pp. 224–225).
2. For a sketch of how an investigation of the compatriot case would go, see Brighouse and Swift (2011).

3. It is an interesting issue the extent to which inequality of opportunity matters because it reflects *systematic* unfairness, and unfairness that is likely to be reproduced over generations. For some kinds of egalitarian, random variation in individuals' upbringings might be a less objectionable source of such inequality than even the properly reformed family.
4. Even though we at no point advocate abolition – indeed the book is written as a *defense* of the family – Gheaus worries that our approach risks alienating and antagonizing readers in a way damaging to the prospects for egalitarian reform. This raises general issues about philosophers' responsibility to anticipate how their ideas might be (mis)understood and (mis)used that we cannot address here. For what it's worth, such opprobrium as we have received has made no reference to our mention of abolition. It has focused rather on the suggestion that parents should occasionally have in mind the way in which even entirely legitimate activities like reading bedtime stories can have the effect of leaving other children at an unfair disadvantage, which has been misunderstood as condemning parents who read such stories. When ideas are prone to that level of distortion, it is hard to see what would be gained by more extensive attention to the possibilities of polemical misrepresentation. Those interested in the opprobrium can find out about it at Crooked Timber (http://crookedtimber.org/2015/05/11/rush-limbaugh-and-bedtime-stories-definitely-not-the-worst-thing-that-happened-last-week/).
5. We consider the case with respect to fair equality of opportunity itself; if justice allowed inequalities of the kind licensed by something like Rawls's difference principle, that case would be more straightforward.
6. Here we follow Sypnowich in using 'neutralist' and 'anti-perfectionist' synonymously. There is of course a considerable literature on the relation between the two, and particularly on whether anti-perfectionism is indeed 'neutral'. We try to sidestep that wider issue.
7. In fact some readers have objected to our cover, variously because the family depicted is American, mono-ethnic, white, heterosexual, patriarchal, and carnivorous. Here we are thinking about the objection that, however wonderful the form of life shown, it is not the state's business to be promoting it.
8. Sypnowich misunderstands our use of Nussbaum's list of the constituents of well-being (Brighouse & Swift, 2014, p. 60), which is invoked not 'to say that children have a right to parents who are best placed to provide them with these goods' (p. xx) but simply to introduce and illustrate the idea of interests.
9. 'Children need the education and upbringing that enables them to understand their own emotional needs and dispositions, regulate their emotional life, and connect emotionally with other people' (Brighouse & Swift, 2014, p. 64).
10. Notice that this is more determinate and specific than the interest in connecting emotionally with other people that we regard as among those developmental interests of children that it is parents' duty to protect and promote.
11. We owe our awareness of this possible difficulty also, and separately, to Norvin Richards (in press) and discussion with Matthew Clayton.
12. Brighouse and Swift (2015) offers further clarification of the specificity of our concerns.
13. For a related view see Weinstock (2016), which we inexcusably came across too late to learn from in this paper.

Disclosure statement

No potential conflict of interest was reported by the authors.

Funding

During the period when he worked on this response, Adam Swift's research was partly supported by a Major Grant from the Spencer Foundation for a project on Faith Schools: Principles and Policies.

References

Benatar, D. (2008). *Better never to have been*. Oxford: Oxford University Press.

Brennan, S. (2014). The goods of childhood and children's rights. In F. Baylis & C. McLeod (Eds.), *Family-making: Contemporary ethical challenges* (pp. 29–46). Oxford: Oxford University Press.

Brighouse, H. (1998). Civic education and liberal legitimacy. *Ethics, 108*, 719–745.

Brighouse, H. (2005). Channel one, the anti-commercial principle, and the discontinuous ethos. *Educational Policy, 19*(3), 528–549.

Brighouse, H. (2006). *On education*. London: Routledge.

Brighouse, H., & Swift, A. (2011). Legitimate partiality, parents and patriots. In A. Gosseries & Y. Vanderborght (Eds.), *Arguing about justice: Essays for Philippe Van Parijs* (pp. 115–123). Louvain: Louvain University Press.

Brighouse, H., & Swift, A. (2014). *Family values: The ethics of parent–child relationships*. Princeton: Princeton University Press.

Brighouse, H., & Swift, A. (2015). Advantage, authority, autonomy and continuity: A response to Ferracioli, Gheaus and Stroud. *Law, Ethics and Philosophy, 3*, 220–240.

Cormier, A. (in press). On the permissibility of shaping children's values. *Critical Review of Social and Political Philosophy*.

Ferracioli, L. (2016). Why the family? *Law, Ethics and Philosophy, 3*, 205–219.

Ferracioli, L. (in press). Procreative parenting, love's reasons and the demands of moraliy. *Philosophical Quarterly*. doi:10.1093/pq/pqx022

Gheaus, A. (2015a). The 'intrinsic goods of childhood' and the just society. In A. Bagattini & C. Macleod (Eds.), *The nature of children's well-being: Theory and practice* (pp. 35–52). Dordrecht: Springer.

Gheaus, A. (2015b). Unfinished adults and defective children: On the nature and value of childhood. *Journal of Ethics and Social Philosophy, 9*, 1–21.

Gheaus, A. (in press). What abolishing the family would not do. *Critical Review of Social and Political Philosophy*.

Hannan, S., & Leland, R. J. (in press). Childhood bads, parenting goods, and the right to procreate. *Critical Review of Social and Political Philosophy*.

Macleod, C. (in press). Equality and family values: Conflict or harmony? *Critical Review of Social and Political Philosophy*.

Rawls, J. (1971). *A theory of justice*. Cambridge MA: Harvard University Press.

Reshef, Y. (2013). Rethinking the value of families. *Critical Review of International Social and Political Philosophy, 16*, 130–150.

Richards, N. (in press). Raising a child with respect. *Journal of Applied Philosophy*. Advance online publication. doi:10.1111/japp.12239

Sypnowich, C. (in press). Flourishing children, flourishing adults: Families, equality and the neutralist–perfectionist debate. *Critical Review of Social and Political Philosophy*.

Tomlin, P. (2016). Saplings or caterpillars? Trying to understand children's wellbeing. *Journal of Applied Philosophy*. Advance online publication. doi: 10.1111/japp.12204

Weinstock, D. (2016). On the complementarity of the ages of life. *Journal of Applied Philosophy*. Advance online publication. doi:10.1111/japp.12204

Weinstock, D. (in press). For a political philosophy of parent–child relationships. *Critical Review of Social and Political Philosophy*.

Index